Happy Families

Happy Families

How to Protect and Support Your Child's Mental Health

BETH MOSLEY, PhD

ROWMAN & LITTLEFIELD
Lanham • Boulder • New York • London

Published by Rowman & Littlefield
An imprint of The Rowman & Littlefield Publishing Group, Inc.
4501 Forbes Boulevard, Suite 200, Lanham, Maryland 20706
www.rowman.com

86-90 Paul Street, London EC2A 4NE, United Kingdom

British Library Cataloguing in Publication Information Available

Library of Congress Cataloging-in-Publication Data

Names: Mosley, Beth, 1975– author.
Title: Happy families : how to protect and support your child's mental health / Beth Mosley.
Description: Lanham : Rowman & Littlefield, [2023] | Includes bibliographical references and index. | Summary: "This honest and accessible guide provides parents with practical advice on the common issues that impact children's mental health—such as anxiety, low mood, and difficult behaviors—and empowers them to make simple changes that can lead to dramatic improvements in their child"— Provided by publisher.
Identifiers: LCCN 2023055536 (print) | LCCN 2023055537 (ebook) | ISBN 9781538190333 (cloth) | ISBN 9781538190340 (epub)
Subjects: LCSH: Child mental health. | Child psychology.
Classification: LCC HQ772 .M678 2023 (print) | LCC HQ772 (ebook) | DDC 649/.1—dc23/eng/20240111
LC record available at https://lccn.loc.gov/2023055536
LC ebook record available at https://lccn.loc.gov/2023055537

To my three children and all they have taught me about love and courage.

Contents

Part 1
Children's Mental Health:
Why is it important?

Part 2
Difficult Feelings:
The good, the bad, and the ugly

Part 3
Anxiety:
How to stop it controlling your child's life

Part 4
Low Mood:
How to get your child back

Part 5
Help:
The secret to giving and getting

Disclaimer

This book is for general information purposes only and is not targeted to readers' specific circumstances. It should not replace the advice of the reader's own physician or other mental health professional. We recommend that readers consult a medical professional in matters relating to health (whether mental or physical).

The author and the publisher do not accept responsibility for any adverse effects individuals may claim to experience, whether directly or indirectly, from the information contained in this book.

Organizations or websites mentioned in this book as a potential source of information does not mean that the author or the publisher endorse any of the information they may provide or recommendations they may make.

All stories in this book are composite, fictional accounts based on the experiences of many individuals, and any similarities to any real person or persons are coincidental and unintentional.

Introduction

The task of being a parent is huge, and that is on a good day when life is going well. It can feel impossible when things in your or your children's lives are not going to plan. The emotional highs and lows of parenthood are like nothing else. Biologically, we're programmed to care most deeply about our children—our task is to get them safely to adulthood—so it makes sense that in this endeavor we face great anguish (trying to keep them alive) and joy (to keep us doing it). We love them, nurture them, mess them up a bit (because it's impossible to be perfect), often wanting for them what we didn't have growing up. Simply put, we want more than to see them make it to adulthood (survive); we want them to be the best versions of themselves (thrive).

Our emotional and physical connection with our children is both pure and complicated. As they grow and develop, our role changes—it has to in order for our children to eventually leave the nest. A baby is utterly dependent on us for everything. A toddler relies on us for most things, but also needs us to encourage in them a little safe adventure to learn about the world and other trusted people in it. A child requires a safe platform from which to go to school, be part of a community, learn to read and write, make friends, express ideas and follow rules. An adolescent, developing relationships entirely outside of us, relying on friends to inform their world, needs help to build the knowledge and skills to make decisions and to look after themselves and others, as they begin to understand the often-dark complexity of humanity.

Our children grow physically and emotionally during this time and face massive biological changes. At times, it can feel like they grow away from us and become strangers. This can be painful. Not only are their bodies and brains developing and changing, but their world is, too. Just like us, they will face losses and disappointments. They will have to go through unexpected change (e.g., loss of significant relationships) as well as predictable change (e.g., transitioning to secondary school). They will encounter pressures we perhaps didn't (social media, constant access to world events), but may experience less of some of the things we might have had as children (corporal punishment, delayed gratification, not being able to see everything we wanted to online). We might have mixed feelings about the value of all these things and feel confused about which of these are benefits and which are burdens.

One thing we know for sure is that we do not come to parenthood as a blank canvas. We have our own story that predates our children— our own journey that we're traveling on while bringing them up. We're often doing all this in the context of our developing relationship with our child's other parent, or perhaps a new partner, who comes with their own history, values and approach to parenting and life. No wonder, as parents, raising children can sometimes feel overwhelming!

As we grow and adapt with our children, we might need a little help—from our partners, friends, family, our community, YouTube, perhaps a professional. We could be worried about some of the things our children are having to deal with in their lives and how it's affecting them. We may have noticed their behavior has changed and are not sure how normal this is. We want to do the right thing, but don't know what that might be. We may notice that a challenge with one child is having an impact on another. Or that our relationship with our partner is under strain or breaking down. Perhaps we're bringing up our child/ children without a partner. Or our own difficulties with mental health may be influencing how we respond to, or worry about, our children. It's likely that you're reading this and wondering how to protect your children from these challenges, while also enabling them to manage the demands of life.

In my experience, these struggles are common to all the families I meet with, whether that is at work or in my personal life. Often, it's difficult for parents to know this about other families because we tend to present the best version of our lives to others, not the warts-and-all one. This is often reinforced by the way society communicates through social media, creating additional pressures to perform well as a parent, couple, and family.

Children's mental health is a hot topic, with many stories on the news about young people's mental health deteriorating in recent years. No doubt you'll have also heard, or experienced firsthand, how difficult it can be to get help for your child's mental health. This raises anxiety and frustration for parents who want nothing more than to protect their children from experiencing distress that leads to poor mental health.

Over the years, in my job as a clinical psychologist working in mental health services, I've met with hundreds of parents who have been confused and worried about their children, unsure if their experiences are "normal" or something to "get help" for. They're often afraid that something they've done has contributed to their child's difficulties. The information I share with these families is often life-changing. It gives them the understanding and reassurance they need, as well as practical, evidence-based tools to support their children through tricky times. Through my work, parents discover that supporting their child's mental health isn't as daunting as they may have initially feared, and they are relieved to find there are clear actions they can take to help their child. They often say, "If only we had known this earlier, maybe we wouldn't be here today."

Fortunately, they and their children realize that these are not just tools to manage difficult times; they are also life skills that can help them be the best (though not perfect) version of themselves. These tools assist in navigating the challenging journey of life with a deeper understanding of what it is to be a human being, with real feelings and powerful thoughts.

I'm writing this book for all parents, not just the ones I meet in the therapy room. I believe if I put this advice in one place, as a simple guide for all parents to access, it will answer their questions and enable them to proactively support their child's mental health, both before and when their child is struggling. Wherever you are in your journey, I hope that this book will empower you in the way I'm able to empower those I meet in person.

Despite decades of training, I have not been the perfect parent. I have three children and—as a single parent—have had to learn how to bring them up while dealing with some unexpected traumatic life events. My children have all struggled in different ways and, as such, I have first-hand experience of the difficulties of applying the knowledge (what we know we probably should do) to the reality (what we *actually* do). I've learned the hard way, like many of you reading this book, how to survive adversity. But I got stuck in survival mode, until one day my daughter asked me: "Why are you always worried, Mummy?" At this point I started to question whether surviving was enough for me, for my children. I wanted to be able to stop rushing toward a distant goal of safety, financial security, and the chance to finally relax and enjoy the labors of my life. As a parent, I kept saying, "When this is sorted . . ." or: "We've just got to get through this." Then, as soon as that thing was resolved, something else unexpected and uncertain came along, and I started saying "When . . . then" again. Looking back at photos of my children, I realized that I was so preoccupied with surviving that I was missing out on being in the moment, seeing my children fully and, ultimately, being the parent I hoped I might be.

Other times, I've struggled with the more mundane aspects of parenthood, sometimes spending the whole day desperate to have successfully got my kids into bed so I can finally "relax." I always seem to be so much more in love with my children when they're sleeping than when they are awake. As I try to relax, I feel that familiar pang of regret that perhaps I was too busy getting through the day to show them this love.

My work has often pulled me away and offered more immediate rewards, occupying my mind and skills more fully. It's hard not to fall into a guilt trap here. There are lots of societal and familial expectations of the parent's role. I'm juggling providing for my children financially, getting intellectual stimulation which is good for me, and having a sense of belonging and identity outside of being a parent—but somehow, I feel bad about this—maybe because, secretly, sometimes I prefer work to parenthood. Work is often more straightforward, the fruits of my labor can be more tangible, and I'm more confident that I'm doing a good job at work than I am at home! Despite loving my work, on darker days, when I'm feeling unappreciated, I can unreasonably resent my children (who are likely resenting my preoccupation with work) for not valuing how hard I work for us all to have a better life. Whether you're employed, enjoy your work or not, we're all juggling the demands of life as we bring our kids up, which inevitably creates complex feelings in us, adding to the pressures.

Grappling with all the dilemmas and feelings parenthood was bringing up for me, it struck me that if I didn't apply the things I talk to others about every day, I would end up burnt out and the opposite of what I wanted to be—a good and loving mother, giving my kids, my friends and family the better version of myself. I started to understand that the things that had happened, or the demands on my time, wouldn't be the reason my kids might struggle with their mental health, but the way I responded to those things would be.

Ironically, the pressure to be perfect, to get it all right, was adding to this absent mom. I was physically there, but always caught up in my own thoughts and worries. This might sound familiar, or it might not apply to you at all. Either way, I hope to convey that I'm not just writing this book as a professional; I'm writing it as a fellow parent who gets how tough it can be on the frontline of your own life.

Author Note

Throughout this book, I have used my twenty years of training and experience to bring together a collection of ideas and skills that may be helpful for you as a parent to understand and use. Interwoven in the text, you will find theories and techniques from a number of evidence-based therapies, including Cognitive Behavioral Therapy (CBT), Acceptance and Commitment Therapy (ACT), Dialectical Behavior Therapy (DBT), Behavioral Activation Therapy (BAT), and Interpersonal Therapy (IPT).

The evidence base for these therapies comes from them being used as an entire program, largely delivered by a trained professional. In my work I have found that parents and young people have found it helpful to learn certain skills that come from different parts of these programs. I am sharing these with you as the families I have worked with have found them helpful. This is not in a bid to help you become your child's therapist, but rather to provide you with a range of tools that might help you communicate with your child and support them when required. Each parent and child is unique, so find what works for you and for them.

If you are worried about your child, speak to a healthcare provider or your child's school for advice and guidance. If this book highlights some of your own struggles, again, speak to someone. Life is complex; we all have experiences that have wounded us. We may be living in a situation that continues to wound us. Healing from these struggles takes time and usually support. Recognizing the difficulty is a critical first step to recovery. Asking for help or support is likely to be an essential part of your journey. It takes courage. I hope this book provides a gateway to understanding more about what we all need, and empowers you to look after yourself in a way that will benefit you, your children, and your family.

There will be opportunities for reflection, as well as suggested activities to complete yourself and with your child. I would recommend that in order to get the most from these you might want to have a pen and notepad, phone, tablet or another device to assist you. Try to look after yourself while reading the book; get comfy. Take care; your children and your life are emotive topics and may bring up strong feelings for you. Read it at the right time, in the right place, at the right pace for you. It is written in a way that allows you to dip into chapters that feel particularly relevant to you or your family. If the book brings things up for you, please reach out for support from trusted others. The signposting at the back of the book is useful to all. Find a resource pack with all the worksheets throughout the book at www.drbethmosley.com.

Where I refer to "parent," this could be any person who cares for a young person in the parent/caregiver role.

PART 1
Children's Mental Health

Why is it important?

Chapter 1

What can go wrong

Olivia's parents sit in front of me. Their faces tell a story of worry and confusion. I can tell they are exhausted and feel alone. They are desperate, grateful to be sitting in front of a professional who—hopefully—can help them. Family life has changed beyond recognition. Home, once a sanctuary, has instead become a place of high tension. Nobody is eating or sleeping properly. Olivia's mom has had to stop working. Family and friends who were so supportive a few months ago now seem to have disappeared. Activities the family used to enjoy together, like sitting down to watch a film or going to the beach for the day, feel like distant memories of another life. Olivia's brother is finding it hard. He thinks about her all the time. He has just started secondary school, but he doesn't want to worry his parents about the things he's finding difficult. He tries his best to manage on his own, but his parents have noticed that he's spending more time alone and not wanting to see his friends. They've started to have concerns about him. "We used to be a happy family," Dad says. "If only we had known how to help Olivia sooner. . . ."

I can feel their love and their despair. Despite this, they've struggled to understand Olivia. They have not been able to protect her from her pain. Most frustrating of all, they've not known how to help.

What has happened to this family to move them from the "happy" family they were to a family in pain and confusion? From picking up this book, you might guess that the family has been struggling with Olivia's mental health.

As we touched on earlier, the mental health of young people has become an increasing concern for everyone in recent years. And rightly so. Mental health conditions (like anxiety and depression) seem to be growing in our children at an exponential rate. In 2021, one in six children aged between six and sixteen had a probable mental health condition, compared to one in nine in 2017.[1] This 60 percent increase is worrying, and further reflected in the 77 percent increase of referrals for children and young people to mental health services in the UK in 2022 compared to 2020.[2]

If these figures were seen in the physical health domain (e.g., if we saw a 77 percent increase in referrals for children to cancer services in a two-year period), we would immediately ask two questions: (1) what's happening to our children and (2) what are we going to do about it?

This book doesn't have all the answers, but its purpose is to provide information to help you in your everyday life, to both prevent and respond to mental health difficulties in your child. It's a book about hope and a guide to get you to the destination you're longing for—being a happy family. I can't guarantee it will be an easy journey, but I can promise you that your love for your child and your dreams for the future will sustain you on your way.

What can go right

Olivia had felt unreachable. Her family went to the darkest of places, but with understanding and support, Olivia returned to them. As expressed in her mother's words to me: "For now, the real Olivia has come back to us and she's looking forward with hope. There will be challenges ahead, but she feels better equipped to recognize and talk about those feelings in the future. The impact you have made on our family is incalculable."

Olivia is now the entrepreneur she dreamed of being. Her parting words will always stay with me: "I will use everything you've taught me in life to help me get through. It has made a huge difference to who I am. I feel like a better person."

For Olivia, the meaning she was able to give to her struggles helped her feel like a better person, illustrating the remarkable power of the human spirit and mind to overcome adversity and use it for good. Just as I helped this family reach Olivia, I hope to help you reach your child. Just as they learned to use the tools I showed them to look after themselves and cope with challenges, I hope to equip you with the tools that will help you adapt to your struggles. As Olivia's family discovered, simple changes can make a big difference. That is what this book is about.

Most importantly, I want you to believe that with the right conditions and knowledge, you have the power to support your child, and while honoring their difficulties, you can build a happy and meaningful life.

☁ Reflection Box

Close your eyes briefly and consider your child(ren). Picture them in your mind. What concerns come to you about where they are with their mental health currently? What concerns might you have for the future? How does it make you feel in your body? Write down these concerns.

Now close your eyes and again, picture your child(ren) in your mind. What hopes do you have for them? How do their strengths contribute to your hopes? How do these hopes make you feel in your body? Write these down.

What do you bring as a parent to supporting your child that you feel is your strength? Write this down.

You may find it helpful to do this exercise again, when you've finished reading the book, to see how your thinking has evolved.

What is mental health?

Mental health is commonly defined as a person's emotional, psychological, and social wellbeing: how we're thinking, feeling, and functioning and how able we are to respond to the stressors in our life. Mental health is not just the absence of illness.

Based on this definition, if I were to ask you, "What's your child's mental health like?" you might frown, look a bit confused and respond, "Well, that depends."

Having met many parents who are worried about their children, I think it's easier to first consider what you care about as a parent. Below are some questions I ask parents when they meet with me.

ACTIVITY BOX

Look at the questions below. While you answer them, consider which areas you think are your child's strengths, and where they may need more support.

* Is my child getting pleasure and meaning out of their life?

* Can they recognize, express, and regulate emotions appropriately for their developmental age?

* Can they recognize the emotions of others (empathy)?

* Do they show an interest in learning both cognitive skills (thinking, learning, and remembering) and social skills (communicating verbally/nonverbally with others)?

* Can they tolerate frustration and follow rules?

* Can they take on social roles (e.g., a student at school, a member of a club)?

* Can they cope with change and manage uncertainty?

Reading these questions, it may have struck you that they seem to be as much about childhood development as they are about mental health. As such, if I were asking you these questions about your child, I would need to know their age and any additional factors (such as developmental disabilities), so I could figure out whether your answers were congruent with what I would roughly expect of a child of that developmental age.

Let's use the example of my seventeen-year-old son, comparing his current behavior to that of his younger self to explore this. When he was two, he might have thrown himself on the floor and cried if he did not get a biscuit. At seventeen, I would expect him to express these emotions of frustration and disappointment quite differently. When he was six, I needed to set up a play date to support him to spend time with friends (with the occasional input from me to share his toys). Now, he meets up with his friends independently. During his early years (aged two to six), unexpected changes would create a big emotional reaction of distress and a degree of resistance. As a seventeen-year-old, unexpected changes are met with a grunt and willingness to move toward problem-solving, as an acknowledgment of accepting the change. Finally, getting pleasure and meaning out of life was different for him as a two-year-old (sitting on my lap, eating his favorite snack, watching *Peppa Pig*) and as a seventeen-year-old (playing rugby with his team, winning).

As you may have identified, your child's strengths in one area might compensate for difficulties in another (e.g., your child's social skills may help mitigate some of their cognitive weaknesses).

When we understand that our child's mental health is intrinsically linked to their development, we learn how important our role is as parents. We also see the impact of factors like our child's temperament, experiences (good and bad), and support/influences around them. Have a look at the activity below to explore this further.

ACTIVITY BOX

It takes a village to raise a child

Your child lives in a world where a number of individuals support and influence them. Write down the key people you think are important to your child's development. This could be family members; friends (yours and your child's); trusted adults, including doctors, social workers, therapists, and community members (e.g., from nursery, school, church, Army Cadets, and Beavers). Some of these relationships might be positive, others less so. We will revisit this in chapter 14 and consider how to encourage strong, trusted connections.

Mental health is not . . .

Mental health isn't fixed and it isn't something we're born with. It fluctuates depending on what's happening in our lives, as well as our skills and capabilities to influence how we're feeling and functioning. Some people find it helpful to think about it being on a continuum, with good mental health at one end and poor mental health at the other.

Mental health is not about being free from all emotional pain. Good mental health still involves times of struggle and suffering. As we will explore throughout this book, our children will experience adversity and loss, and these stressors will impact their thoughts, feelings, and behaviors. Just like joy, experiencing emotional pain and loss cannot be avoided. Emotions are the tools humans use to adapt in our imperfect world, and our children will need help from the important adults around them to help make sense of these emotions and use them to help their bodies and minds.

When our children are struggling with difficult events and feelings, it's natural to ask, "Is this normal, or do I need to worry?" and

"What should I do to help?" This book will uncover the answers to these questions and give you the tools you need to support your children.

Mental illness

Mental illness is a term that explains a range of mental disorders that affect a person's mood, thinking, and behavior. Typically, it would be associated with high levels of distress and difficulties functioning in social, school (work), and family activities. These disruptions to mood and functioning would be disrupted over a sustained period, to the point that the child's age-appropriate ability to function in a range of areas of their life was impaired.

Signs relating to anxiety, low mood, and self-harm will be covered in detail later in the book. In the meantime, here are some clues that might suggest a child is struggling to cope with some of the challenges they are facing and may need more help:

* changes in behavior (high levels of emotion, or a lack of emotion);
* difficulty sleeping;
* not doing things they normally like;
* withdrawing from connection with others;
* not looking after themselves.

Difficulties are more likely if: (1) these changes have been going on for a long time (e.g., weeks/months rather than days), (2) there are a number of these difficulties happening at the same time, and (3) they are having an impact on your child at school, home, and/or their relationships with friends and family. Over the course of this book, we will explore how you make sense of what might be going on in your child's life to explain these changes, and how you can help.

Why childhood and adolescence are important

The body and brain develop most significantly during childhood and adolescence. The brain's growth and development starts before a baby is born and continues throughout childhood up until around the age of twenty-four. It's neither a blank canvas nor a finished piece of work. Genetics and experience work together to support its growth and development, which is fundamental to a young person's ability to move, regulate emotions, learn, and problem-solve. How a young person thinks or feels about their life and how well they can manage the challenges life presents will be influenced by their brain development.

As the body and brain develop most significantly during childhood and adolescence, it's no surprise that this is when they are most sensitive to experiences that can impact mental health.

With 75 percent of mental health difficulties in adulthood starting before the age of twenty-four and 50 percent by the age of fifteen, statistics confirm this. If mental health is the "foundation for emotions, thinking, communication, learning, resilience, hope and self-esteem,"[3] childhood and adolescence are when this foundation is built.

What puts mental health at risk

In order for a child to develop and stay well, both physically and mentally, there are some absolute essentials they require.

Survival needs
They need to have a safe place to live and sleep, nutritious food to eat, fresh air to breathe, and clean water to drink. They need to be able to keep clean, stay warm or cool down (depending on the climate) and have suitable clothes to wear. They also need to be safe from abuse (physical, emotional, sexual) and conflict.

Attachment needs
Children are dependent on an adult to not only meet these physical needs and keep them safe, but also provide them with love through emotional warmth and care. The attachment-emotional bond between parent(s) and child is vital to emotional, psychological, and cognitive

development. According to physician Gabor Maté, within this attachment, the child needs to feel from the parent that they "are precisely the person they love, welcome, and want."[4] Ideally, from this nurturing relationship with their parent(s), they will learn about the world, develop a positive sense of self, and build trust in others to meet their emotional and physical needs. This relationship should also provide a safe place from which to learn how to stay safe, play, and follow appropriate rules. Essentially, within this relationship a child learns what it is to love and to be loved.

Social and cognitive needs

Children need opportunities to feel safe in their communities and social world and grow their knowledge. In these communities, they have the chance to build relationships that can help them develop and grow their emotional and social skills and build meaningful connections with others.

With both attachment and social needs, a child needs to have a sense of agency, so that they feel that they can positively influence the world around them. All these factors, to varying degrees, promote healthy child development and protect mental health.

Risks to mental health

Situations or events that put these physical, emotional, and psychological needs in jeopardy (either by not having them in the first place or by being at risk of losing them) will create stress in a child's brain and body (described on page 144). This increases the risk of disruption to a child's healthy development and their mental health.

Children who experience socioeconomic disadvantage, harsh parenting, discrimination, bullying, any type of abuse, parental mental illness, exposure to domestic violence, living with someone who abuses alcohol or drugs, loss of a parent through divorce, death or abandonment, and conflict (such as wars and disasters) are more vulnerable to difficulties with their mental health due to the additional stressors they might experience. For many of these children, the support they have in their life will protect them from some of the impact of this stress.

Some children might experience an unexpected or stress-inducing event that disrupts the stability and order they rely on to feel safe and loved (e.g., an accident, parental divorce, moving house or school, the arrival or departure of a sibling, physical illness). During this time, a child may need more reassurance and care. Some children may struggle for a short while as they adapt to the change, but others may take longer to adjust, and need additional support.

COVID-19 has had an impact on many young people's mental health because of the changes it forced on their lives. Among many things, loss of control and not having the structure and support of school and meaningful activity will have contributed to feelings of distress and unhappiness.

Many children are reporting that the everyday pressures of life— schoolwork, exams, juggling the demands of a digital world—are creating stressors that are contributing negatively to their mental health.

Your unique child

No two children are the same. Our child's uniqueness is made from their individual genes, biology, and the environment in which they grow up. These factors will contribute to their biological, psychological, and social growth. This in itself is a huge topic, so I've touched on some key points that I believe you'll most want to know:

* Our child's experience in the womb can influence how the brain develops: the mother and baby's bodies are physically connected in the womb, so the mother's biological stress response affects the development of her baby.

* There is an increased risk of developing difficulties with mental health if one of our parents did. This risk is not just

influenced by genes, it's also influenced by other biological factors and the environment a child grows up in.

* Some children's temperaments can influence how they experience the world.[5] Your child may be particularly sensitive, making it difficult to settle them when they were a baby. They may be more reactive and sensitive to change and their environment. If you've identified that your child is more vulnerable to distress, you might also notice that it's harder to support them when they are distressed. If you have more than one child, you might recognize this is a unique characteristic for one of your children, compared with the other(s).

* Children with an intellectual disability, learning difficulty (e.g., dyslexia, dyspraxia), neurodiversity (e.g., attention deficit or communication disorder) face more challenges as they grow up. As such, their development may not follow the same trajectory as neurotypical children. This can increase their risk of struggling with their mental health, especially if they are not provided with the right support or adaptations to their environment.

* Children with chronic health conditions, including asthma, are more likely to experience a mental health disorder. Reduced attendance at school and a higher chance of bullying contribute to this.[6]

* Young people who identify as LGBTQIA+, an ethnic minority, or another discriminated group are at higher risk of poor mental health for myriad reasons that include increased chances of discrimination, social isolation, and rejection.

As you might expect, the more vulnerabilities and experiences of adversity a child experiences, the greater the probable impact on their mental health.

What is neuroplasticity?

Don't panic if you believe your child has experienced some difficult events in their life, if there is a family history of mental health difficulties and/or you see them as having a more sensitive temperament. The wonderful thing about the brain is that it's flexible and adaptable throughout our lives. It can build new connections and learn new ways of relating to others and ourselves—this is neuroplasticity. During childhood and adolescence, the brain is particularly flexible and great at learning new things. As parents, we have a double opportunity to support our children to learn these new skills and brain connections, and also develop these areas in our own brains.

What's happening to our children?

Headlines like "COVID-19 pandemic triggers 25 percent increase in prevalence of anxiety and depression worldwide"[7] confirm that mental health is hugely impacted by the stressors that individuals are exposed to and the resources they can deploy to adapt to those stressors. We can safely say that anxiety and low mood are natural responses to the uncertainty, huge changes, and additional stressors the pandemic created for most people.

When we go back to the unsettling figures at the beginning of the chapter and ask what's happening to our children, perhaps these increases in mental health difficulties reflect the world we're living in—one with increasing stressors that undermine mental health.

What can we do about it?

If you let that question sink in for a minute, it can make you feel pretty helpless as a parent. At the end of the day, we know our children will experience stressors we can't control, and that societal pressures, economics, and popular culture will contribute to these stressors. So, what does this actually mean for us? What can we do about it?

Firstly, being aware that there is not necessarily something "wrong" with your child when they are struggling is important. Your child's struggles may be a natural response to the challenges they are facing in their increasingly complex world. Secondly, the greatest power we have as a parent, regardless of their mental health status, is our relationship—our bond with them. Lastly, how we understand our children (their thoughts, feelings, and behaviors), how we relate to them, how we make them feel, and how we support and guide them can all contribute massively to their ability to adapt and cope with the challenges they face.

This book will help you understand and relate to your child better, support your child's wellbeing to buffer against the impact of stress and provide support and guidance to your child when they are struggling with their mental health.

SUMMARY

→ Supporting the mental health of all children is a priority because of the increasing numbers of young people across the world developing mental health disorders.

→ Mental health mirrors a person's emotional, psychological, and social wellbeing: how we're thinking, feeling, and functioning and how able we are to respond to the stressors in our life. The tasks of child development influence mental health.

→ Mental illness describes mental disorders that affect a person's mood, thinking and behavior to the point that they experience extreme distress and their ability to function in social, school, and family activities is significantly reduced.

→ The body and brain develop most significantly during childhood and adolescence. This makes the brain especially sensitive to experiences that can impact mental health.

→ Protective and supportive environments in the family, at school, and in the wider community protect mental health.

→ Adversity, unexpected stressful events, and a range of factors unique to your child's makeup influence mental health.

→ Parents are an integral part of their child's development and are therefore well placed to:

- support the wellbeing of their child to buffer against the impact of stress;
- provide support and guidance to their child struggling with their mental health.

Chapter 2
The must-dos

As parents, we're in a prime position to help prevent our children from developing mental health difficulties. If they do struggle, we can provide them with the support and guidance they need to recover and build good mental health. In this chapter, we will explore the Wellbeing Abacus, which explains how stress impacts wellbeing and what we can do to protect our children and ourselves against these stressors on a daily basis.

Mental wellbeing

Mental wellbeing refers to how we feel (about ourselves, others, and our lives) and how we function (experiencing positive relationships, having some control over our lives and having a sense of purpose). It's influenced by what's happening in our lives (including the stressors described in chapter 1), as well as our own skills and capability to influence how we feel and get on with life.

An important element of wellbeing is our ability to feel and understand the full range of emotions, both the ones that make us feel good (e.g., happiness, pleasure) and the ones that make us feel bad (e.g., sadness, regret). When we enjoy good mental wellbeing, we're likely to spend more time experiencing emotions that make us feel good and doing things that give our life meaning and purpose.

What can we do to support wellbeing and protect mental health?

Research tells us there are five things we should do that have a positive impact on wellbeing (feeling good and functioning well):[8]

* connect with others;
* physical activity;
* take notice;
* keep learning;
* be giving.

Over the course of the book, you'll find these five ways to wellbeing woven into the pages. I have added two additional areas—sleep and nutrition—between physical activity and take notice as they are both key components to mental health and something we as parents can monitor and influence.

Understanding the importance of these seven areas is valuable because not only do they support wellbeing, but difficulties in these areas could help us identify mental health struggles. We will take a look at each of the seven areas briefly, before exploring how Olivia's mental health struggles (introduced in chapter 1) were reflected in changes in these areas.

1 Connect with others

Meaningful, positive relationships are integral to humans. They support our wellbeing in a number of ways:

* physiologically (they help reduce our stress response and improve immune function);
* psychologically (they help us regulate our emotions and provide opportunities for learning and guidance); and
* socially (they give us a sense of belonging and help us feel like we're contributing to the wellbeing of others).

It's no surprise, therefore, that the biggest predictor of wellbeing is positive and supportive relationships with others. It's vital for their wellbeing that children feel loved and cared for, and have a sense of belonging and opportunities to connect with others, whether it's family members (parents, siblings, extended family), trusted adults (school staff, youth workers), and/or friends. Importantly, safe and nurturing relationships (even just having one of them) have been found to protect young people from some of the physiological and psychobiological impacts of adverse childhood experiences.

Bruce Perry[9] and countless other eminent child doctors and therapists describe the importance of the child's attachment—the quality of the bond—with their primary caregiver. In this book, I do not cover attachment theory specifically, but instead use the principles of attachment throughout.

In simple terms, the research tells us that having parents (and other adults) who communicate acceptance and availability through emotional warmth (affection; kindness; giving guidance, time and attention when needed) is protective of wellbeing and mental health, even in the face of childhood adversities. In contrast, having parents who communicate rejection through low emotional warmth and high control or neglect (low emotional warmth, low control), or parents who are overprotective, is linked to lower self-esteem and psychological inflexibility. Both self-esteem and psychological flexibility (being able to stay in contact with the present moment, despite difficult emotions, and acting in a way proportionate to the situation that is consistent with your values) are key determinants of wellbeing.[10]

As described in chapter 1, relational stress through exclusion (e.g., discrimination, bullying), disruptions to important relationships (e.g., loss of a loved one, parental separation) or conflict within relationships (e.g., arguments with parents/friends) can lead to difficulties with mental health.

When people are struggling with their mental health, it can be more difficult for them to communicate with, and connect to, others. Likewise, it can also be more difficult for others to communicate and connect with them. When I meet with parents, this is their biggest concern. "What is going on with my child? I want to be able to connect with them and help," they say.

When a child is anxious or low, they often feel misunderstood, meaning the quality of their relationships reduces, yet this is when they need these positive relationships the most. As a parent, understanding how strong feelings, anxiety, or low mood may be affecting your child (helping you see beyond the surface), knowing how to connect and how best to advise them, can make the difference between your child's difficulties growing or being resolved.

② Physical activity

We often view physical and mental health as two separate things, but the more advanced studies in both fields become, the more evidence there is that the two are unequivocally intertwined. Stress has a physical impact on our bodies—it affects our immune system and our inflammatory response among other things. It makes us want to take physical action to get away from the threat (see fight-flight-freeze on page 144).

Today's lifestyles are both stressful and sedentary. This poses a problem. Moving our bodies is the single most effective way to help process the stress chemicals that build up in our system, while producing feel-good chemicals that give us a boost and protect our physical and mental health (see page 156 for more on this). Whether our children are experiencing stress or not, they are often not getting enough opportunities, or lack the motivation, for physical activity. We will be exploring the mind–body link and how to support the body to improve low mood and anxiety as well as general wellbeing.

③ Sleep

Good-quality sleep is essential for our bodies to heal and recover from the activity and stressors of the day. Without sufficient sleep, our brain's threat response (amygdala) is more sensitive. Because of this, if we or our children do not get good sleep, we will be more irritable, focus on the negative, feel more anxious, and find it hard to remember things and concentrate. Just as our sleep affects how our body copes with stress, high stress levels can disturb our sleep. This can create a vicious cycle with lack of sleep exacerbating difficulties with anxiety and/or low mood, and anxiety/low mood further affecting sleep (see page 152 for more on this).

Adolescents are more likely to have difficulties with sleep because of changes in their circadian rhythm (the hormones they release make them tired later in the day—see page 287).

It's common to experience sleep difficulties at one time or another, particularly in childhood and adolescence. Persistent poor sleep (difficulties falling asleep and/or staying asleep) is likely to affect wellbeing and may also be a sign that your child is struggling with their mental health. Often, especially with adolescents, we might not be aware of sleep struggles. You can, however, easily check in about sleep—asking in a kind and curious way (so they don't think they are in trouble). Use the Wellbeing Abacus worksheet (resource pack) as a conversation tool.

Providing young people with information about sleep and some simple changes to sleep habits can make a big difference (see page 219 for more help).

4 Nutrition

Our children's food habits can be a source of potential joy (enjoying sharing food and eating together) or stress (the pressure of eating the right foods for healthy growth, enough variety, and enjoying mealtimes). We may often worry whether our children are eating enough of the right stuff and not too much of the wrong stuff. A bit like digital technology (which we'll look at in chapter 3), we have a huge range of options with foods, and some of the things our children are drawn to are the things we worry might be unhealthy.

What we eat and when we eat have an impact on our health and wellbeing. Generally, the patterns of eating we get into and the range of food we eat can impact our brains, both in the short and long term; this can affect our mood, attention, ability to learn, energy levels and sleep.

Getting stressed about what our children do and don't eat can itself be counterproductive, so knowing that small changes in the following areas can make a big difference will hopefully help reduce the pressure you might feel in this area.

Nourishment
Modern-day eating in developed countries typically gives us access to a huge range of food. Many of these foods are highly processed and lack the nutritional nourishment that supports the micronutrients in our blood and the microbiome in our gut (the balance of bacteria and microorganisms). Processing foods takes them far from the original natural ingredients they came from, meaning they are often packed full of fuel and additives (sugar, fats, calories), but lacking in the nutrients and fiber our bodies need (think of a skin-on potato, compared to a bag of potato chips). Fiber helps the energy the food gives us last longer and supports our gut health. This is important for health and wellbeing.

David Rex, a specialist dietician, suggests that when encouraging our children to eat, the most important thing is to encourage variety (rather than get stuck on bad versus good foods.)[11] Providing access to a range of different fresh foods and modeling eating these foods ourselves encourages: (1) a more nourishing diet and (2) children to eat foods they might initially be reluctant to try.

Food–mood rollercoaster
What we eat and when impacts our blood glucose, which affects our attention, irritability, and energy levels. Eating regularly throughout the day (three meals and a snack in between) is important in maintaining a steady trickle of blood glucose. Missing meals leads to crashes in blood glucose levels, which can impact concentration, energy levels, and irritability (HANGRY)! I've noticed the biggest arguments in my household are just before dinner or a meal, particularly when everyone comes in from school. When children do not eat during the school day (perhaps due to anxiety), the impact on learning and their

increased sensitivity to stress can be a real worry for parents. If your child is about to engage in a more demanding activity—even if it's a difficult conversation with you, doing a chore or completing some homework—hold in mind when they've last eaten. Their tolerance and concentration might be influenced by this. Timing and a snack can make a big difference between something going well or an escalation in distress.

Brain health

There are many micronutrients that have an impact on the brain. Four of these are magnesium, iron, vitamin D, and omega-3 (see table below). Due to the modern-day diet, our children can be deficient in these four micronutrients, which can impact their brain health (mood, learning and attention). The foods that have high levels of these nutrients are ones we might find difficult to include routinely in our children's diets, in which case you may consider a supplement. Talk to your family doctor or pharmacist to get their input on what's best for your child (or you, if you believe you might be deficient).

Our brains are made up of 60 percent fat, so it therefore makes sense that we need the right types of fats for them to work effectively. Our diets tend to be low in omega-3 fats (which largely come from oily fish). Some research has found that high-quality omega-3 supplements taken over a consistent period of time can in some cases reduce ADHD symptoms, improve attention, behavior, sleep and, for the poorest readers, even reading.

Brain Micronutrients	Brain Health
Magnesium (Whole grains, leafy greens, beans, peas, nuts and seeds)	Many children are magnesium-deficient, as they do not eat enough magnesium-rich foods. Magnesium deficiency has been linked to behavioral difficulties and anxiety in children. Consider a good-quality magnesium supplement (suitable for a child). Speak to your family doctor or pharmacist.

Brain Micronutrients	Brain Health
Iron (Red meat, beans, dried fruit, nuts)	Iron is vital for the production of red blood cells. Deficiencies can lead to tiredness and fatigue. Adolescent girls have a higher iron demand and are at more risk of iron deficiency (anemia). If you're worried about this, you can speak to your family doctor, who may suggest an iron supplement.
Vitamin D (10 percent from food like oily fish, 90 percent from skin being exposed to sunlight)	Vitamin D is very important for bone health; it helps the body absorb calcium. Some research is exploring its impact on mental health. Ensuring our children have adequate access to the outside and a vitamin D supplement (10 micrograms) in the autumn and winter helps avoid deficiencies.
Omega-3 (Fish/seafood, rapeseed/flaxseed oil)	Anti-inflammatory and anticoagulant (reduces blood clots), omega-3 is an important part of our diet for brain health. If your child does not eat oily fish, a high-quality supplement can serve as an alternative. If your child has any health issues, discuss with your family doctor before supplementing.

As we will discover later in the book, feelings of anxiety and low mood can interfere with appetite. For a small number of young people, excessive control around eating can be a way to cope with stressors and pressures. Sensory sensitivities can also contribute to restricted diets. Observing changes in our children's eating can be a useful indicator that they are struggling with their wellbeing.

5 *Take notice*

Focus is a real challenge for young people today, as it is for adults. The world is full of stimulation and competing information and often we divide our attention between multiple activities. This is especially true with the use of screens, with children often using multiple screens at one time for different purposes (e.g., playing a game on one screen while watching YouTube or messaging friends on another). Providing opportunities to be focused in the here and now gives the brain a chance to rest rather than constantly thinking about what's happening next, or what has already happened. Regular mindfulness practice—"paying attention on purpose, in the present moment, and nonjudgmentally"[12]—has been shown to have a positive impact on wellbeing for some people, but not all.[13]

Mental health difficulties involve our thoughts. When struggling with mental health there is a tendency to focus on the negative and ruminate (to go over and over) on the things that are bothering us. Getting better at taking notice and learning how to break this cycle are key components of the evidence-based therapies used to treat mental health difficulties.

6 Keep learning

Learning provides opportunities to develop knowledge and skills, which can lead to achievement, a sense of mastery, independence and, ultimately, improved wellbeing. As our children grow and develop, they have a huge number of things to learn about themselves, others, and the world. Children's experiences at home, school, and in general offer opportunities to do this learning.

Stress affects the ability to learn, as the part of the brain that is triggered by stress shuts down the part of the brain we need for thinking and processing new information (see chapter 4). If our children experience stress, they may find it more difficult to engage with learning and gain a sense of achievement. This becomes a vicious cycle, adding further stress and impacting both children's attainment and school attendance.

A child who struggles in areas of learning because of difficulties with concentration, coordination, organizing themselves, understanding other people's points of view, or their experiences of stress, can be exposed to repeated failure in the learning environment. This can be damaging to a child's sense of self and ability to engage in learning, reducing their opportunities for developing skills to help compensate for these difficulties.

We can help our children build a growth mindset by providing opportunities for them to experience success, which reduces their distress, and instead encourages them to reframe failure as an opportunity to learn.

-🔆- The mouse trap: Learned helplessness

The following example contains references to animal testing, which you may prefer not to read.

Research into mice has demonstrated the power of repeated failure in the face of inescapable and uncontrollable distress. The term "learned helplessness" emerged from early research in this area. Let's look at a study of two mice to explain this.

Mouse 1 is put in a cage where the floor delivers a mild electric shock that is uncomfortable for the mouse. He explores the cage. When a gate opens, he escapes. The next time he is put in the cage and the shock-floor is activated, he explores and quickly exits via the gate when it opens.

Mouse 2 is put in the same cage. He initially explores, but no gate opens. Instead, he experiences the discomfort until he is removed from the cage. This is repeated. When he is eventually put in the cage and the gate is opened, he does not attempt to escape.

Mouse 1 had the opportunity to escape from the uncontrollable stressor. Mouse 2 neither had control nor the opportunity to escape. His best chance was to conserve energy. Eventually, even when presented with the opportunity to escape, he did not take it.

> ☁ **Reflection Box**
>
> Are there times when your child's repeated failure has led to them giving up? How do they deal with this frustration and pain? How has this affected their approach to other tasks?
>
> Have you ever experienced this yourself? What small things can be done to support your child experiencing their own success (both in terms of practical and moral support)?

As illustrated in this lab experiment, our approach to a challenge comes from the experience of being successful. The same is true for resilience, which comes from doing hard things and being successful (not repeated failure). Encouraging our children to be brave enough to try new things or to try again if they struggled the first time is important. However, the role of adults in ensuring the task set is achievable for that child and, if necessary, providing them with just enough support to do the task if required (psychologists call this "scaffolding"), is more important.

If your child is struggling in an area of learning, it might be because they have a skills deficit, not a will deficit. If so, make it a priority to help them to build this skill alongside providing them with the opportunities to feel successful. This will build their confidence and love for learning. Sometimes, our children may need help from a specialist professional in an area they may struggle in (i.e., a speech and language therapist for communication difficulties, or an occupational therapist for coordination difficulties).

7 *Be giving*
When we look after each other, we all do better. Doing nice things for other people—something as simple as a warm smile and a "thank you"—releases feel-good neurochemicals. Even seeing someone else doing something kind has the same effect on our biology. Recent research in this area has shown that simple acts of kindness lead to

bigger improvements in alleviating depression and anxiety than two other well-evidenced techniques! David Cregg and Jennifer Cheavens, the psychologists who led the study, believe this is because it helped people feel more connected to others.[14] They also found it had the biggest impact on those who tended to have more difficult personalities.

As a parent, you spend every day giving constantly to those you care for. In this act of service, giving might not feel quite so positive, especially as the tasks we do are generally mundane and taken for granted. Often, the spirit in which we do things is as important as the act itself. Perhaps if we do these things as if they are acts of kindness, rather than what they've become—duty—not only will we feel better, but we might get more appreciation and reciprocity from those around us. (I'm going to try this at home!)

ACTIVITY BOX

Challenge each family member to twice in a week complete three acts of kindness in a day (big or small)—things that make others happy. Make it fun by creating an ideas list with your kids (they might not know the simple things they could do for you that would feel like acts of kindness). Describing the acts of kindness at the end of the day (something you could do at a mealtime or before bed) can reinforce a sense of gratitude and positivity (see the Simple Acts of Kindness activity worksheet in the resource pack).

The Wellbeing Abacus

Paying attention to what's happening in these seven domains of wellbeing can be helpful in these ways:

* alerting us when the stressors and pressures in life might be getting in the way of doing things that are good for our wellbeing; and

✳ helping us think about how we can proactively support our
   wellbeing by doing more of the things that count.

I've developed the Wellbeing Abacus as a useful tool to teach your
child about the seven ways to wellbeing (see the Wellbeing Abacus
activity worksheet in the resource pack).

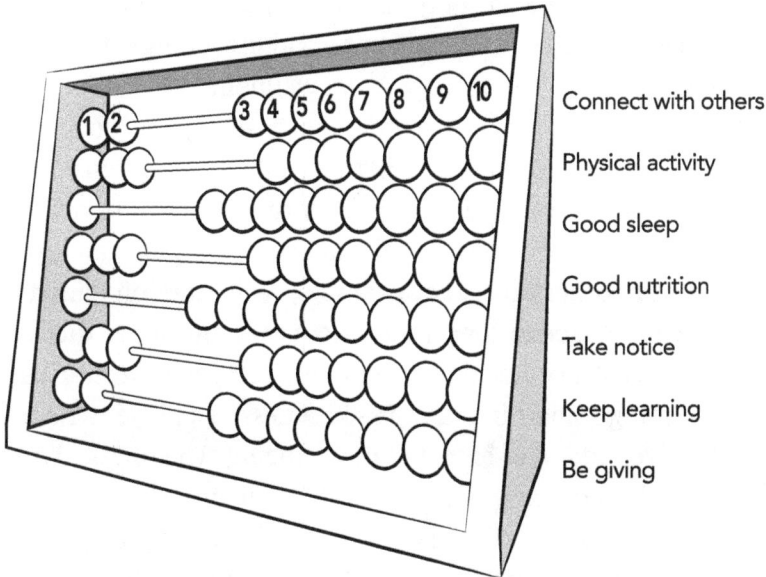

Connect with others

Physical activity

Good sleep

Good nutrition

Take notice

Keep learning

Be giving

The Wellbeing Abacus

Think of each line of the abacus being a continuum from 1 to 10, with
10 being the best we might be doing in that area, and 1 being the
worst. Consider how things are going in each of these seven areas at
any given time and how this might be impacting wellbeing. It's important to note that we can go up and down the continuum—it's not fixed
and can be altered by experiences, thoughts, and feelings.

   If you or your child are struggling in an area with a low score,
consider (a) what's contributing to this difficulty, and (b) how, by
taking action, waiting for the passage of time, or changing of circumstances, the score can increase.

Domino effect

You might notice that as one bead on the abacus slides down, another bead naturally does too. For example, yesterday I had a bad night's sleep. This had a knock-on effect for the rest of the day. I missed breakfast, found it really hard to concentrate at work and felt I couldn't take on a new project, even though it was something that interested me. I was also more irritable with my children, creating conflict and strain in my connection with them. Because I had low energy, I decided not to go to the gym. As a consequence, my wellbeing throughout the day dropped. Thankfully, after a good night's sleep, my abacus beads moved up the following day and I felt my wellbeing (my sense of enjoyment of the day and being able to get my tasks done) improve.

In the same way, one bead on the abacus sliding up can lead to an improvement in other areas. For example, when my son joined a new basketball club, his bead for physical activity went up, as did his connection to others (he made new friends and felt part of a team) and his sense of learning something new. His kindness to a player who fell and hurt themselves added to his sense of wellbeing. The physical exertion meant his body was tired, so he also slept well later that evening.

Our abacus beads fluctuate constantly throughout the day, depending on our experiences and how we're responding to them.

Top Tip: Scaling Questions

Quite often when we ask our children about their day, or an area of their life, their answer may be fairly nondescript (i.e., "OK," "Fine") or all-or-nothing (i.e., "The worst ever" or "Brilliant"). It can make it feel quite hard to have a meaningful conversation or understand what's going well or not so well for your child. Solution-focused therapy uses scaling questions to help people who might be feeling overwhelmed to put a number (usually out of 10) to their situation or feeling. This does several helpful things. Firstly, it helps a person step back to get a bit of perspective. Secondly, by breaking down the difficulty, it gives you ways to talk to help consider realistic solutions to the problem, or just get to know more about your child.

A scaling question involves asking someone to rate out of 10 how something is going or how strong a feeling is. So, for example, with the Wellbeing Abacus sleep bead, I might ask my child: "If 1 is the worst sleep ever and 10 is the best sleep possible, what number would you put your sleep at the moment?" You can use the same scaling question to consider feelings as well as situations. You don't have to use numbers. Instead, you could draw a line on a piece of paper (with "worst" at one end and "best" at the other) and ask them to put a mark on the line where they think they are.

Next, you can ask more scaling questions to help gain more understanding of what's going on for your child and also encourage positive change. So, let's say my son replied he was a 5 for sleep. I could ask him, "What stopped it being a 4?" He might then explain he's doing something that helps his sleep. He might say, "It helped not going to bed too early, or I would have been lying there awake for ages; that would have made it a 4." To help him think about what could be different to improve sleep, I might ask, "What makes it a 5 and not a 6?" He may then tell me: "Well, all my thoughts are spinning around my head, making it difficult to fall asleep. If I didn't have those busy thoughts it could be a 6 or a 7." We can now think collaboratively about how to encourage the things that are helpful and resolve some of the things that are unhelpful. In the resource pack, the Wellbeing Abacus worksheet gives examples of scaling questions you can try.

The impact of stress

It's not just how we spend our time and what we do that influences the beads on our Wellbeing Abacus. It's also the stresses and adversities we experience in our lives. As described in chapter 1, chronic (ongoing) and acute (one-off) stress impact our physical and mental health.

Because of this, while we're enduring difficulties, or in response to them, our abacus beads will probably slide down the continuum.

The most important thing to understand is that this drop is a natural response to our feeling difficult feelings (sadness, anger, loneliness, fear) in response to these stressors. Understanding and sitting with these feelings will enable us to make important changes in our lives and resolve situations that are creating distress. If we can't resolve them, we can at least make sense of them and consider, "what now?" The difficulty comes if what we do:

1. does not lead to a change in the situation that is causing us distress; or
2. might protect us from the specific situation that is causing the distress (e.g., cutting off painful feelings, not seeing friends, etc.), but may have a negative knock-on effect in other areas of our life (e.g., being unable to feel joy, increased loneliness).

The trigger for Olivia's distress (head back to page 11 to revisit this) was persistent bullying, both at school and online. Let's look at the box below to see what happened to Olivia's wellbeing beads as a result of this chronic stress.

Olivia's Story		
Olivia's Wellbeing Abacus scores	Before	Now
Connect with others: Olivia previously enjoyed spending time with friends, but since the bullying started, in order to protect herself from being hurt (physically and emotionally), she has stopped interacting with her friends. Being more emotionally reactive, she won't cooperate with adults, leading to disagreements with her teachers and parents and behavioral reprimands at school and at home. She no longer feels she makes a positive contribution to her community.	7	2

Olivia's Story		
Olivia's Wellbeing Abacus scores	Before	Now
Physical activity: Olivia used to play team sports. She loved basketball. Her difficulties with her friends mean that she has stopped going to basketball club. She generally does less physical activity, as she does not want to do things with her family either, meaning she spends a lot of time sitting or lying down doing no exercise (sedentary).	9	3
Sleep: Olivia has never been a great sleeper, but things have worsened. She can't go to sleep at night because when she tries, all the thoughts about worst-case scenarios pop into her head, making her feel sick and causing her heart to race. She uses her phone as a distraction, visiting chat rooms into the early hours of the morning and reaching out to strangers for comfort. Because of this, it's difficult to wake her in the morning.	6	1
Nutrition: Olivia used to enjoy eating a range of foods, but her appetite has changed. She goes a long time between meals. Lack of regular food and disturbed sleep means she relies on energy drinks to keep her awake in the afternoon.	7	3
Take notice: Olivia has a curious side. She used to like to question things and paid attention to the world around her. She noticed things more when she was out with friends or family and enjoyed taking photos of scenes she thought were special. Lately, Olivia feels like she has been in a permanent "fog." She's stopped enjoying the taste of food and her attention seems to be taken up with negative thoughts.	7	1
Keep learning: Olivia used to enjoy school some of the time, and particularly liked learning coding in computer studies. Now, she struggles to concentrate in lessons and spends more time in class feeling anxious about break and lunchtime. She has started to fall behind in her classwork and has lost confidence in her abilities. She used to enjoy learning new tunes on her guitar, but she has lost the motivation to pick up her guitar.	7	3
Be giving: Olivia used to like to help her grandma mow her lawn. She also enjoyed helping her friends when they were finding things tough with a helpful text message. Olivia now finds it hard to think about giving or being kind to others. She feels so consumed with her own thoughts and feelings, she struggles to consider what other people might be thinking and feeling and how she might be able to help them or be kind to them.	7	2

Olivia's change in behavior, as demonstrated in the drop in Wellbeing Abacus scores, tells us something important about what's going on in her world. It gives us clues that Olivia is experiencing some distress, affecting her ability to enjoy and get on with life. With this information from the Wellbeing Abacus (as illustrated on page 37) Olivia's parents could look at the "signs of mental health difficulties" on page 17 to help them work out how much to worry about Olivia and what level of support she might need.

The meaning behind the behaviors

Looking at the seven different domains on the Wellbeing Abacus only tells us about the behaviors. It does not tell us the meaning behind the behaviors or the purpose/function of them. As parents, our children's behaviors are what we notice first, which can sometimes be a distraction from what's going on underneath the surface. How these behaviors make us feel (e.g., angry, scared) can drive our response to our child, and we may unintentionally react in a way that reinforces the feeling or worry behind the behavior.

In Olivia's case, her behavior told people she was out of control, did not respect school and family rules, and was reluctant to invest in relationships. She was perceived as having an issue with authority, but the feelings underneath this behavior were fear, the pain of rejection, and loneliness. As a result of the bullying, her defense to protect herself from further pain of rejection was to withdraw from others and lash out at them. Although this might have protected her from contact with the bullies, it had a knock-on effect on the other key areas that contributed to her wellbeing and did not enable her to get the support she needed. Furthermore, the adults around her responded based on what they *thought* her behaviors suggested she needed (e.g., boundaries and consequences). In doing so, this unintentionally reinforced her feelings of inadequacy and rejection.

> ☁ **Reflection Box**
>
> Think about some of your child's behaviors you find more difficult. What feelings do they create in you? What might be hiding behind these feelings and behaviors?

Connecting with the distress

Before Olivia can start to see an improvement in her wellbeing, we (as the adults around her) need to:

1. understand what's causing the distress, and, if possible, stop it (in this case, cyber- and in-person bullying);

2. help Olivia to feel her painful emotions associated with the bullying, understand what these feelings mean for her ("I hate feeling rejected and alone") and clearly communicate these emotions to supportive others, so that her needs for belonging and connection can be met.

If Olivia feels safe again, and has the support and understanding from her parents and other adults in her life, she is then in a good position to consider, with the help of her parents, how small changes in the seven areas on the Wellbeing Abacus can lead to improvements in her wellbeing.

Simple ideas to help Olivia's beads move along the Wellbeing Abacus (which, cumulatively, could make a big difference to her mental health):

1. *Connect with others*
   Talking with and feeling understood by her parents, having a trusted adult at school to get support from.

2. *Physical activity/keep learning/take notice*
   Going to the gym with her uncle and cousin a few times a week (giving her a chance to exercise), learning new skills in the gym, and through the training opportunities focus on the here and now.

3. *Sleep*
   Following the sleep hygiene tips on page 219.

4. *Nutrition*
   Eating more regularly and not drinking energy drinks (which were contributing to problems with sleep).

5. *Be giving*
   Doing one simple act of kindness a day, like making her mom a cup of tea or helping unpack the shopping.

Until Olivia received support to understand her feelings and share what was going on in her internal world, she felt unreachable to her parents.

By feeling understood, Olivia was able to reconnect with her parents (and they with her). Together, they were then able to identify small, manageable changes to help her have a healthier sense of control of her life and improved wellbeing.

Parenting: The tricky bit

The keys to your child's wellbeing can sound deceptively simple when written down like this. The reality is, just as Olivia was to her parents, our children can often be an enigma to us and unreceptive to our best attempts to guide them. Their behavior can be enraging, exhausting, and remarkably confusing. No other person in my life has ever led me to feel the rage all three of my children have managed to innocently incite in me over the years.

Let's not forget, each of us was once a child. Our childhoods were full of the things described on pages 19 to 21, which have influenced who we are today. These experiences give us strengths and weaknesses and inform our expectations and hopes for our current family. We must remember to be kind to ourselves as parents; it's a tough job, and feeling worthless drives feelings of parental stress and loneliness.

Stress doesn't just affect our children; it affects us too. As you're reading this, you may be grappling with the daily stressors and pressures of life. Perhaps you have additional concerns about money, relationships, work, discrimination, or your own physical health or mental health. If we're living with adversity and stress, our focus on keeping ourselves and our children fed, warm and safe can make it hard to prioritize our relationship with them. We can be there in body—but not in spirit. When I look back at photos of my children, I realize with great sadness that I was often so preoccupied with surviving that I was missing out on being in the moment, seeing my children fully and ultimately being the emotionally available parent I hoped I might be. I reflect on this with compassion, as I was doing my best with the resources I had, and at the same time I recognize I can do better.

As parents, and humans, we're not perfect. We all have our own stories. But it's important to know we don't have to get it right all the time. Just enough of the time. The chaos of life can often distract us from a simple truth: what our children want is more of us—our love and affection. This is one of the biggest predictors of a child's happiness, along with how we manage our own stress.

The principles I share in this book will help you be more attentive to your own needs as a parent, so that you can be more attentive to those of your children. I acknowledge that the contexts we live in, including the social, economic, and health inequalities many of us face, can sometimes make this feel impossible. That for many the complexities of past experiences and current daily challenges, which will often feel outside of an individual's realm of control, mean none of this is simple. But I anticipate that in reading this book, if you apply some of these principles to yourself, that in itself will create a change in your child and your family. Remember: showing someone the way is often more powerful than telling someone the way.

It can be lonely: Find your cheerleaders

When I was left alone with each of my three children as new babies, I was struck by the loneliness and level of isolation I felt. My daily routine and connection to others disappeared. The world seemed to be getting on without me and I did not feel part of it. The magnitude of the task of looking after my baby felt overwhelming. Time took on new meaning. Night and day merged into one. I often think these times were both the most connected with another person I've felt, yet simultaneously, the loneliest moments of my life.

From an evolutionary perspective, we're not meant to parent in isolation. Our ancestors parented in communities and had the support of a multigenerational tribe to manage the stressors and demands of raising children. It was a collective task, filled with support and contact with others.

My best advice to you is to find your cheerleaders: the people who pick you up when you're down, who make you believe "you've got this" when you're about to give up, and hold hope for you when yours is wavering. The people who kindly tell you the truth when you're struggling to see it. Invest in these relationships. Be honest with these trusted people and let them be your cheerleaders. Cherish them. Let them cherish you. Believe you're good enough to warrant them. If you can, find someone to whom you want to be a cheerleader. Giving can be as good as getting.

If you feel you have fewer cheerleaders and more referees, critics, or bullies in your life (life is full of those, let's be honest), make it a priority to find cheerleaders. You might discover that those you usually turn to—friends, family, work colleagues, a professional—will quickly and happily take up the role. A cheerleader could even be an influencer online who gives you the boost you need when days seem hard. The more cheerleaders you have from different walks of life, the more opportunity for learning, growth, and the ability to weather storms. Most importantly, the more energy you'll have to be your child's cheerleader.

ACTIVITY BOX

Having insight into our daily lives and how they fluctuate in the seven ways to wellbeing can be helpful. Throughout the book, you'll be able to use the Wellbeing Abacus to help you build activities into your family's daily routines and rituals that support these areas (see page 158 for an exercise to help you do this with your child). In the meantime, go back to the Wellbeing Abacus on page 37 and complete the two exercises below.

1. You

Think about a day when things went well for you. Go through each domain and rate yourself out of 10 on each of the seven areas. Now think about an event in your life that has created distress for you. Go through each domain and rate yourself out of 10 for each domain during that time. What elements of your life were missing or suffered during that time? What parts of your life did you manage to maintain and were supportive of your wellbeing?

2. Your child

Think about your child this past week. Rate them on each domain. In which areas are they scoring lower? Which areas are they scoring higher? Consider what could be impacting each area and where you feel they need more support.

Over the course of this book, you'll learn about the importance of connecting with others—how you can build stronger connections with your children, find ways to communicate with them when they are struggling and teach them how to communicate with others when things are going well, not so well and when in crisis. You'll explore the mind–body link and how physical activity can support the body to improve low mood and anxiety, as well as general wellbeing. You'll identify when poor sleep might be a sign your child is struggling with their mental health. You'll discover a range of different simple activities that will show you and your child how to practice the art of taking notice and being in the here and now, to not only build self-awareness, but also to positively influence how you relate to yourselves and others. You'll harness your child's neuroplasticity and need to keep learning, and will unlock the tools to help your children learn about their emotions, what's important to them (their values), how to overcome problems, and what to do when anxiety or low mood get in the way. You'll obtain the information and tools to provide you with what you need to give a little and often to the best effect.

These seven ways to wellbeing will help you to identify how you can support your child's wellbeing, so you can not only protect your and your child's mental health, but also notice where you or your family life might be compromised.

SUMMARY

→ Good mental health and wellbeing is how satisfied we feel (about ourselves, others, and our lives) and how we're functioning (experiencing positive relationships, having some control over our lives, and having a sense of purpose).

→ There are seven steps you can take that have a positive impact on wellbeing: connect with others, physical activity, sleep, nutrition, take notice, keep learning, be giving.

→ Using the Wellbeing Abacus to explore with our children and pay attention to what's happening in these seven domains of wellbeing can be helpful in:

- giving us clues when the stressors and pressures in life might be getting in the way of our child doing the things that are good for their wellbeing;

- helping us think about how we can proactively support our child's wellbeing by doing more of the things that count.

→ Being a parent is tough, especially when we're experiencing stress and pressures ourselves. Prioritizing these areas for ourselves is important in giving us the best chance to support our children.

→ Building a network of supportive people (your cheerleaders) is an important part of looking after yourself so you can have the resources to be your child's cheerleader.

Chapter 3

Screen time— how much is too much?

We're at the swimming pool. I'm sitting on the side with my thirteen-year-old daughter. "Mum—someone's messaging me right now; I know it—I've got a feeling. I really need my phone!" I can see her spiraling, fighting the urge to leave the pool, go to the lockers, and check her phone.

"Don't worry about it, you can check it later," I say casually. The truth is I had exactly the same thought about my phone, but it wasn't a message I was worried about: it was work emails. I seem to have become obsessed with knowing that I'm on top of my email inbox.

"No, really, Mum, I have to check it—it might be important!" she protests, agony on her face.

I feel it. I could have missed something important, rings through my mind. I need to keep us both in the moment. "Let's see who can do the biggest jump in the pool?" I say. With no hesitation, I run away from the thought of my emails and jump. Cold water shocks my system. As I come up for air, I feel an explosion of water next to me and I know she's jumped in too. For a few blissful moments, we will be immersed in another world where our brains will forget about our phones. We have both temporarily escaped our addiction.

Our children are growing up with digital technology and screens as an intrinsic part of their world. As adults and parents, we probably find ourselves equally dependent on this technology. It's what we rely on for work, learning, entertainment, and social connection. We may consider that digital technology and screens have made certain elements of our lives easier. But at what cost? How do we realistically ensure that the benefits of this ever-evolving digital asset do not cost our children their wellbeing?

Your questions about screen activity are likely to be along the lines of: How much is too much? Can screens be used positively? Why is gaming addictive? What is the impact of social media use on mental health? If, as covered in chapter 2, how we spend our time impacts our mood and activity levels, does how we use digital technology do the same? This chapter explores these questions.

How much is too much?

As a parent, you'll be well aware of the friction screen time can create within the family. Our children may seem to want to exist in an entirely virtual world and it can be difficult to know (a) how much to allow our children to engage with this world, and (b) how to influence or control the level and type of engagement.

I've lost track of the number of times I have planned activities (e.g., "It's beautiful out there, let's go to the beach for the day!") and my children have responded with disgust and resistance as their preference is to stay in their bedrooms engaged in their alternative universe (whether that is gaming, watching videos, and/or socializing with friends). In these moments, my heart sinks and rage builds as I battle to convince them to put down their devices in exchange for the guarantee of "a good time." ("We'll have ice cream and hot dogs—it will be fun!") The promise of "a good time" is not enough; I resort to threats of turning the Wi-Fi off. They sulk for the journey and look at me like I'm the cruel killer of fun. I can't remember it being like this when I was a kid. I'm sure we all jumped for joy when my parents suggested a trip out! I recall boredom in childhood spurring my imagination, forcing me outside and providing opportunities for the contemplation of life. I remember being compelled to write poems or song lyrics as I filled my time of youth tuning into the radio, tie-dying dungarees, and fantasizing about a boy who did not even know I existed! It was a better world, I think, gripping the steering wheel, trying not to explode with: "I don't know why I bother!"

Invariably, they do have "a good time" as they become absorbed in the day (although I still catch the odd wistful look into the horizon, as if thinking of a distant lover). On the way home, I'm filled with joy. "See, I told you it would be fun; so much better than being stuck in your room all day." When my ten-year-old replies, "Yes, it was fun, but I could have watched 14.2 episodes of *The Simpsons*," my heart sinks. Measuring time in TV episodes. I open the front door. Off they run, back to their bedrooms, reunited with their devices with not a second glance back at me. "Where have I gone wrong?" I ask myself. The truth is, I rely on screens to keep the peace in my household and to quietly entertain my children when I'm busy managing life, leading to this love–hate relationship, and the dilemma: "Is it possible to have my cake and eat it too?"

Surprisingly, the recurring questions of "what are screens doing to our kids?," "how much is too much?" and "are increases in mental health difficulties caused by social media?" have not been conclusively answered. Research is still in its early days and government-commissioned reports resort to a noncommittal solution: Doing anything too much ends up not being good for you, so "families should try to find a healthy balance" between normal activities and screen time.[15]

Researchers at the University of Oxford completed a study on the impact of technology use on 300,000 adolescents in the UK and the USA and found that technology accounted for a tiny 0.4 percent of adolescents' wellbeing. "Comparatively, eating potatoes has nearly as negative an effect, and wearing glasses has a more negative effect on adolescent mental health than screen use,"[16] purports their eye-catching headline. The researchers are clear: using statistics this way won't answer our questions in this area. It's more complex. And I would agree: the dilemmas I face around serving my kids potatoes for dinner and the use of technology do not seem comparable.

As a parent, I feel I'm fighting a losing battle. Screens seem to be woven into every part of life. How do I harness the good and avoid the bad, not just for my children, but also for myself?

A few points that highlight the challenge:

* Screens include all kinds of devices such as television, smart phones, tablets, computers, video game screens (monitors) and smart watches.

* There are an infinite number of ways you can engage with each of these devices: completing online work, communicating with friends, recording exercise, looking up a recipe, gaming, taking photos and using video-sharing platforms.

* We can use screens to engage in concurrent activities. Children are increasingly "multi-screening" as a part of everyday life. Typically, this involves browsing social media on one device while also gaming, watching content or learning on another.[17]

Based on these realities, research suggests we need to move away from focusing on how many hours our children are spending on their screens and instead focus on what they are spending their time doing.

Active versus passive

If our children are spending their time in what we call "active use" (such as messaging their friends, playing online games with their peer group, creating a TikTok or doing something that is age-appropriate and requires active participation), these activities are generally considered better for wellbeing. In contrast, more passive use of screens, such as scrolling through Instagram or TikTok for long periods of time, is linked to a decrease in wellbeing. Naturally, excessive use of either type of engagement can negatively impact the parts of life that we know are critical for health and wellbeing.

This information is helpful to know, but can still feel too simplistic in the face of how we're using our devices:

* ✳ "My son is gaming with his friends (active use) while scrolling through a video platform (passive use)." Where does this fit—is this good or bad, or does the good cancel out the bad and make it neutral?

* ✳ "My daughter is messaging friends but getting caught in a cycle of negative commentary or experiencing bullying." This is active use, but you can see it's having a negative impact.

* ✳ "My child has uploaded a TikTok they enjoyed making. They've been happy with all the likes, but a negative comment has resulted in tears." Again, as a parent, you can see and feel the pluses and minuses.

Inevitably, as we live out these experiences in our families, we think, *I wish my child could experience life without this additional complication!*

> ☁ **Reflection Box**
>
> Write down your thoughts on screen time and social media. What do you like about them? What do you find more difficult or dislike about them? What does digital technology add to your life? What does it take from it?

To help you with these questions and dilemmas, I'm going to spend the rest of the chapter using the Wellbeing Abacus from chapter 2 to guide you through this complicated territory. How we use screens to either facilitate or disrupt each of the seven areas of wellbeing is likely to have an impact on our children's development, levels of distress and, consequently, their mental health.

Connect with others

Our children will use their devices in various ways to feel socially connected to others: through messaging, group-text chats, video calls, and online gaming. They may also use platforms like Instagram and TikTok to feel connected to their friends, make new friends and keep abreast of the latest trends that will help them feel a part of youth culture and a specific community with which they might identify.

As described in chapter 2, we cannot underestimate the fundamental importance of social connection (particularly for adolescents). Research into the use of digital technology and social media highlights how much young people value this medium to enable them to stay connected with friends and family, as well as make new friends.[18] Not only does it allow them to spend time together when they are physically apart (e.g., watching a film together while communicating via messaging chat), but many young people feel it also provides opportunities to express their thoughts and feelings more freely, especially in anonymous spaces.

Digital technology provides opportunities to make new friends and connect with others who share similar interests, which can be particularly helpful for young people who fall into a minority group or have a specialist interest not shared in their immediate peer group. Living in a fairly rural part of the UK, students I meet with often express how finding an online group of others who they might identify with (e.g., LGBTQIA+ community, other neurodiverse young people) can be life-changing, giving them a safe place to express their ideas, explore their identities, feel less alone and increase their sense of belonging. Young people also describe being able to seek out and receive support from others while online. This could be their friends or supportive organizations.

Social disconnect: The tricky bits

Just like in-person relationships, the way our children connect with others online comes with risks. Cyberbullying is one.

Cyberbullying

Online bullying can take many forms, depending on how young people are interacting online. It can happen through messaging apps, social media platforms, or online gaming. It can include targeting a child by making negative comments to or about them through messaging, or posting negative comments on their social media posts. It could involve creating fake profiles, taking photos and digitally manipulating them, or posting images or videos that might be embarrassing or humiliating.

A high proportion of young people are likely to have experienced some kind of cyberbullying. Girls and young people from minority groups (e.g., LGBTQIA+, BAME, disability) are more likely to have experienced it. Professor Andrew Przybylski,[19] a respected researcher in the area of screen-time use, stresses that it's important to understand not just if a young person has experienced cyberbullying, but how often and how severe it is, to help consider its possible impact on the young person's wellbeing.

Cyberbullying rarely occurs in isolation. Typically, it's linked to face-to-face bullying. Therefore, most often it's an avenue for a child already experiencing bullying to be further victimized. This can increase the potency of the experience of being bullied. In chapter 2, we saw how Olivia was bullied at school and online. Olivia was not able to escape the bullying when she was at home because it continued on her phone outside of school and in the evenings, which increased her distress. As parents, remaining curious about changes in our children's behavior and providing them with opportunities to share their experiences of feeling bullied, whether "offline" or "online," is more likely to lead to putting an end to the bullying.

Every child is different, and their resources to cope with some of the elements of the online world can vary. Some young people may be more impacted than others by a negative comment online, depending on their vulnerabilities, relationships and other stressors that may be present in their lives.

Our children may not be able to manage their own behavior as well as we would like, as they are developmentally out of their depth. I noticed my younger son losing control of his behavior toward his peers when playing high-adrenaline games, often shouting aggressively at others, sometimes swearing when he wouldn't usually. I've also experienced my daughter getting involved with negative chat cycles which I worried might hurt another young person's feelings—yet she seemed oblivious to this. In both these instances, I'm aware my child's behavior might be experienced as bullying by those they are interacting with. Just like when they are not on their screens, our children are having to learn what is and what isn't appropriate behavior. There may be times when they are swept up in the energy of their virtual worlds, or do not directly witness the impact of their behavior on others, leading to challenges and sometimes distress in both themselves and others. Although we may not be able to do it all the time, staying connected and aware of how our children are behaving online gives us the opportunity to support their development in this area.

As with other social skills our children are taught, providing clear boundaries around acceptable behavior and encouraging feedback and opportunities to develop these pro-social skills is often in our gift. Taking an approach that allows collaborative conversations with our children around the value and purpose of these boundaries and behaviors is likely to be more helpful than just asserting them. In doing this, we ensure we're curious about the context and create space for our learning about some of the cultural nuances of their world (e.g., I wrongly assumed a skull emoji was negative, when it's used as a way of conveying laughter).

Support versus co-rumination

Relationships can be supportive, but also destructive. We have all experienced a conversation with a friend, where you start off feeling bad and end up feeling worse. Somehow, your friend's worries, anger and frustrations have reinforced your own, and you're now distressed about things you hadn't even considered at the beginning of the conversation. The potential for these unhelpful in-person interactions is lower, because in moments of high distress we often have to wait until we meet with an appropriate person to have that conversation; typically our distress would have abated somewhat by then. Having our phones with us at all times and knowing we can contact others at any time of the day or night means that at that peak moment of high distress, we can reach out immediately. Sometimes we might reach out and get back much-needed support and help to reduce our distress, someone who will validate our feelings and provide some sound advice (e.g., "Don't message them now; wait until you feel less upset"). Sometimes we reach out and what we get back can escalate our distress through co-rumination (feeding each other's negative thoughts) and influence our actions with bad advice (e.g., "They've asked for this—post that photo now!"). As we explore later in chapter 14, if our teenagers are reaching out to other teenagers, particularly those who are distressed or unaware of their advice's impact, they are more likely to get the latter than the former. In these vulnerable moments our children might turn to online platforms, where unhealthy and sometimes harmful methods to cope with their distress might be suggested. Worryingly, our children's online exposure to self-destructive ways of coping with distress are often high, leading to a youth culture where these ways of coping with distress are normalized and sometimes minimized.

This is where our relationships with our children are so important, as they provide the balance that might be missing in these interactions. If we're available to them when they want to rant about an injustice, our children might come to us before they reach for their phones. If they get an unhelpful response from a friend, or online platform, they might seek us out instead of getting stuck with their distress. If our children believe we're genuinely interested in their world, without us rushing to black-and-white thinking ("This is why I hate phones, just ignore them") or judgment ("You're wasting your time and energy"), they might give us more opportunities to influence it. Helping our children work out which friends or adults are helpful to turn to in a crisis and which people or places lead to increased distress may also help them become more discerning about who they turn to for support and guidance.

The same is true for disturbing content. Around 50 percent of twelve-to-fifteen-year-olds report having experienced some form of negative online experience. Reassuringly, nine in ten children aged eight to fifteen would tell someone if they had seen something worrying online. For all children, the most likely person is a parent. Older children are more likely to tell a friend than younger children.[20] Ideally, we don't want our children to see these images or be contacted by strangers and we can set up restrictions to limit the possibility. However, if our children accidentally or deliberately see violent, disturbing or pornographic content or images of self-harm, knowing they can turn to us to have constructive conversations that help make sense of what they've seen and how it makes them feel is more important than our own distress that they've seen it at all.

Pursuit of perfection

The online world provides lots of opportunities to look at other people and their lives, which may be the curated version they want us to see. Our children scroll at high speed through thousands of images and videos of a mixture of celebrities, influencers and peers. Often filters and image-manipulation have been used to project the preferred image. Our children might do the same in their posts. We might. This can lead to something described by the Royal Society of Public Health as "compare and despair." It's hard not to measure your own self, your own life, against these often-enhanced images.

This creates several unhelpful pressures. Firstly, it can set unrealistic expectations about how one should look, the shape of one's body and the type of emotions one should experience to be happy (e.g., feeling popular or desired). Secondly, in order to be part of this world and accepted in it, our children may find themselves posting images that enhance their own face, body and emotions, projecting a false image of who they are, relying on affirmation and "likes" of this augmented version of themselves. When these images are "liked," it adds to a pressure to present something they may not actually be or feel. This cycle can lead to young people sitting with me, crying tears of desperation, as they explain: "Nobody understands the real me. I feel so alone; everyone thinks I'm so together, but actually, I'm falling apart." It's a cruel and fickle world. The very same followers who liked their feed can just as easily dislike it or make a throwaway comment (often devastating to the receiver), if they perhaps reveal a bit too much of their "real" self—getting an angle wrong or looking less desirable in another image.

Seeing your child caught in this trap is excruciating. You want to shout, "It's not real; they are all faking it! Stop caring about this pointless stuff and it won't hurt." But teenagers are biologically programmed to care about this stuff (see chapter 14). A lack of empathy from us is likely to make them feel worse. We also fall into the same trap, though perhaps less extreme, as we scroll through other people's feeds and feel twinges of irritation or envy at their apparently fantastic lives, responding with our own posts which might inflate the positive version of our own lives.

The best way we can help our children, and ourselves, is to be interested and accepting of the "real" them (and us). It takes a lot of energy and hard work to maintain a persona. Authentic relationships are liberating, as they enable the bits of us that even we don't like to be accepted by others. If we can see beyond the surface of our children's behavior, we give them the gift of our acceptance and love for who they are, not who popular culture pressurizes them to be. At the same time it is important to not be dismissive of their online world and some of the choices they might make to present themselves. Some of the social media platform tools give young people the confidence and creativity to share their experiences and view of the world. Sometimes the use of a filter may act as a shield, helping a young person be more honest about their internal world, as they share authentic content about their struggles with others.

I remember a magical moment in my career that changed things for me. I was providing a parent workshop in a school. The parents all looked a little hopeful as they sat in front of me, but also tense, as if waiting to be made to feel like bad parents. I was having a particularly difficult time as a parent and instead of presenting myself as the perfect psychologist, ready to bombard them with "how to get it right," with radical honesty, I told them stories about my daily battles of knowing what to do in theory, and what I actually did in reality. The relief in the room was palpable. Parents laughed, nodded, felt understood. I could tell they also felt hope. When I finished, to my surprise, they applauded me. One parent stood up to speak: "Thank you for being so honest. If you, with all your years of training, find it hard as a parent, it gives us all hope that we can do this." I was reminded that how I make people feel is often more important than what I say.

Previously, I had worked so hard to always appear faultless, to not let the stuff slip out I didn't want others to see. From that day forward, I endeavored to be as honest as I could with my friends and work colleagues about not being perfect, not getting it right. Not in a bid for people to feel sorry for me or excuse me, but instead to allow more honest conversations. I quickly learned how powerful this was; it stopped everyone having to pretend, to deny their difficult feelings. I could have more real interactions with people, which would lead to feelings of validation, followed by resolution of the genuine problems.

The same was true in the anxiety workshops I ran at schools. One teenager, seeing another student whom they thought "had it sorted" sharing that their sleep was ruined by worry about how others viewed them, immediately felt relief from the feeling: *I'm such a failure for struggling like this.* Unexpectedly, for the self-conscious teenager in this safe space, they discovered that their honesty earned them affection and respect.

Understanding that even the most together-looking people have moments of doubt and difficulty can encourage others to believe in their moments of doubt or difficulty; they are not broken. It also means we're more likely to be kinder to those who might not, on the face of it, seem to need the kindness.

Our children and teenagers are on a path of discovery, trying to work out who they are in an increasingly complex world. If we can help them make sense of how they feel, their thoughts and what they do, we will also provide the space and context where they can turn to us without feeling judged or told off. We can help them make sense of what's real and not real, in others and themselves (digital or otherwise). We can accept that this is the world our children are in; it will create both joy and pain, relief and pressure. This frees us up to consider how we can provide a safe space to turn to when they feel overwhelmed, have made a mistake or have been hurt by something. From this position, we're more able to guide them to make better choices and be less reliant on their esteem coming entirely from this source. Through this, we can also encourage them to develop skills of critically evaluating what they see online, as well as staying safe.

Balanced opportunities for in-person and digital social connection

We want our children to develop good social skills and pro-social behaviors in all contexts. We also want to protect them from destructive interactions that could negatively impact their view of the world and of themselves. We should encourage and support our children's opportunities to develop these social and relational skills in both in-person and digital worlds, with adults around them to guide their behavior.

We can support these opportunities by encouraging our children and teenagers to meet up with friends in environments where they have adults at hand to constructively guide them (even if it involves us picking their friends up to come over). I've been surprised by how willing my daughter and her friends are to share their dilemmas when I'm curious, interested and balanced in my responses. I find that even when they meet in person, they seem to rely on their phones to communicate and spend their time together. I often wonder if the phone serves as a security blanket, protecting them from more authentic conversations, or if they've not yet acquired the skills to spend their time together without their phones.

Don't underestimate the value of your child being around you when you interact with your own friends in person. They can learn a lot from seeing you demonstrate these skills. Being fully present with our friends and our children, putting our phones out of sight, can encourage more authentic and meaningful conversations.

Many children lost out on the opportunity to spend time with others in person during the pandemic. For some youngsters, this impacted the development of their social skills, as well as other important areas of development (e.g., language, coordination, sensory). These young people may need additional support from parents, school and other professionals (e.g., speech and language therapy, occupational therapy) to help develop skills and confidence in these areas.

> ☁ **Reflection Box**
>
> Think about your child's time connecting socially. Write down the practical things you can do to encourage more *positive* social connection in your family. Write down what changes in your approach could help protect against the *disconnect* described above.

Physical activity, sleep, and nutrition

Research has attempted to explore the impact of screen time use on behaviors that are linked to both physical and mental health, including sleep, physical activity, and nutrition. Not surprisingly, the research suggests that there is an association between increased screen time use and reduced physical activity, reduced quality of sleep, and an increase in calorie consumption. Furthermore, some research suggests that young people struggling with anxiety or depression spend more time on their screens.

These are associations, rather than causes. We cannot say that increased screen time causes these difficulties. The researchers describe a chicken-and-egg scenario: we don't know which comes first—poor sleep or increased screen time use. Do young people who are more sedentary spend more time on screens because they are doing less of other activities? Do young people struggling with anxiety or low mood, which disrupt sleep and other activities, turn to their screens as a way to cope? In other words, does increased screen use *come from* the initial difficulties, rather than increased screen use *causing* the difficulties? Does a young person struggling with anxiety or low mood engage with their device in a way that might increase anxiety or low mood (e.g., spend more time co-ruminating or focusing on negative information)?

Spending huge amounts of time on any single activity (even activities that are good for us in moderation) will be detrimental to other important activities. If I become engrossed in a good book and sit for eight hours reading, I might not engage fully in other parts of my life. I won't speak to my kids, cook them dinner, go on a walk, and I might stay awake until 2 a.m. just to get to the end!

Until the research becomes more sophisticated, we have to rely on common sense. If we know good-quality sleep, opportunities for physical activity, and eating a balanced diet are good for wellbeing, ensuring we create opportunities for our children to build these things into their lives and reduce the barriers to accessing them is likely to be helpful. This can be through small, simple changes that enforce good habits and protect from some of the more distracting or negative aspects of digital technology. For example, not having smart phones in bedrooms overnight when we know our child might be prone to waking up and checking messages, eating snacks and meals away from the screen, protecting times of the day for physical activity—even if it's five minutes of dancing around the living room or a walk round the block.

There are useful elements of digital technology that can support us in the areas of physical activity, sleep and a balanced diet—from smart watches that track physical activity and reward movement to apps that support sleep through relaxing, breathing exercises and soothing stories, or recipes that encourage healthy and regular eating.

As explored further throughout the book, changes in our child's sleep, activity levels and eating can be indicators of our child struggling with their mental health. In my experience, a child's exposure to conflict, loss, loneliness, unexpected changes, or problems at school is likely to have the biggest impact on a child's wellbeing. The way they use screens may be an attempt to cope with the feelings that come from these experiences and may inadvertently contribute to further difficulties. Therefore, asking "What is happening in my child's world?" (at school, with their relationships, how they feel about themselves) is probably more useful than focusing on "How much screen time should my child have?"

ACTIVITY BOX

What small changes can you make in your family routine to encourage balance in the areas of sleep, physical activity, and eating? If your child struggles in any of these areas, write down some of the other things that are happening (or not happening) in their life that could explain why screens have become such an important part of their daily routine.

Take notice

If we're preoccupied with our digital world, or constantly distracted by messages, we may find our awareness of the world around us goes down. If, while walking, we're reading the news on our phone or responding to a message, we may miss a beautiful sunset, and not notice our feelings or the physical experience of being alive. If our child walks into the room with an expression of unhappiness when we're dealing with a work email on our phone, we might find we miss the cue to notice what's going on for them, and lose an opportunity to connect in a meaningful way. Dopamine is all about the future, and getting so much of it from our devices (and other preoccupations) could prevent us from fully experiencing the moment. It can introduce unexpected stressors in moments that would be better protected for fully engaging in "doing" activities, or spending time with those we care about (e.g., an unexpected message, newsfeed, or email that pops up on your phone can distract and trigger the fight-flight response, just as you're enjoying another activity or about to go to sleep). Screens run the risk of distracting us and taking our attention away from what's important in the moment.

When our young people (or we) engage in something pleasurable like a video game, the brain releases something called dopamine, a neurotransmitter, which provides a feeling of pleasure. It's the excitement of what's to come. It gives us energy and hope and makes us feel motivated.

Our evolutionary ancestors would have relied on dopamine to ensure that things that aid survival grabbed their attention (e.g., a gazelle on the horizon, berries on a bush, a potential partner). The rush of dopamine creates the energy and motivation to pursue these things, not out of fear, but out of desire. To take the required risks and tolerate the discomfort of exertion, dopamine gets you fired up until you reach your goal.

The future versus here-and-now

Dopamine is not the only neurochemical that gives us pleasure. Serotonin, oxytocin, and endorphins do too—these important neuro-chemicals help us enjoy the moment and feel satisfied with life. We tend to activate these when we're present in our experiences (e.g., being physically and emotionally close to others, or engaging in cre-ative activities that use our bodies and minds).

Lieberman and Long (2018) describe in detail the delicate balance between dopamine (drive) and these here-and-now (satisfied) chemicals. Their book, *The Molecule of More*,[21] highlights how important it is to provide opportunities to use dopamine wisely so that we don't get addicted to always wanting more; to ensure that we give the here-and-now satisfied neurochemicals the opportunity to provide the balance we need to protect our mental health and wellbeing. We need both here-and-now and future neurochemicals to experience meaningful lives, but what we do and how we pay attention can hugely influence the balance between the two.

When the body produces increased levels of dopamine, it deactivates the production of the here-and-now feel-good neurochemicals. (For our ancestors to hunt, they needed the "satisfied" neurochemicals switched off, or else they wouldn't bother to go through the exertion to chase the gazelle down.) It's similar to a seesaw (see the diagram on the next page): when the here-and-now chemicals are activated, dopamine production is deactivated. This helps us relax and enjoy the moment. Being motivated and enjoying life requires the delicate balance of these two systems. The system can be unbalanced by our experiences. If we're immersed in constant dopamine-driven activities, we can find it hard to transition to enjoying the moment and feeling satisfied with life. Likewise, if we get stuck in the here-and-now with intense negative thoughts and feelings, this can deactivate our motivation and energy to resolve a problem.

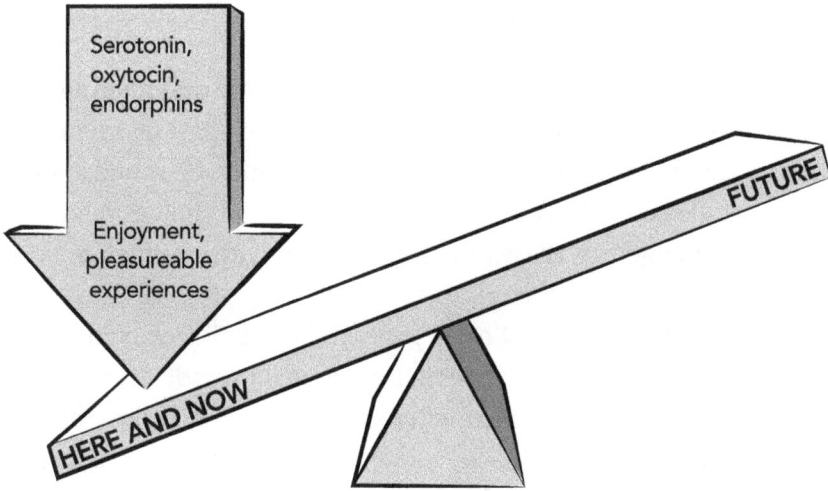

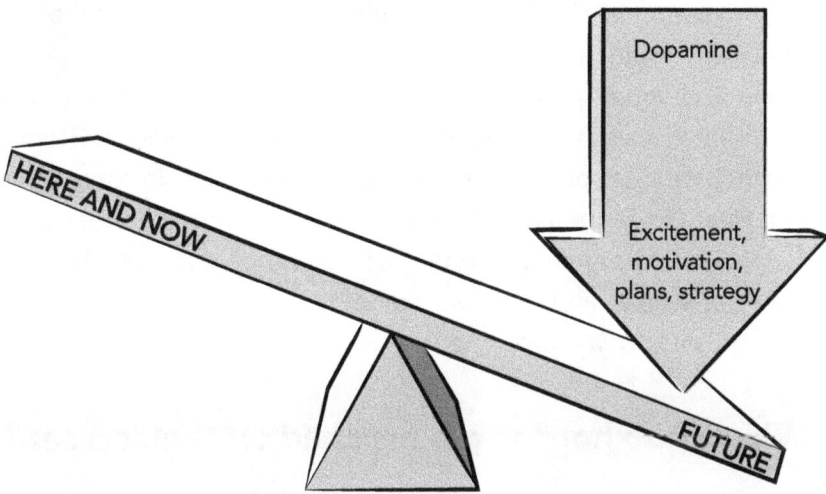

Thinking about how we consciously encourage these here-and-now opportunities and deliberately paying attention to what we're doing may involve putting devices away during activities. As suggested in the Top Tips Box (page 71), it involves us creating routines that protect certain times of day or activities from the distraction or allure of our devices. Our children will need more help with this because their self-discipline and impulse control is likely to be less developed than ours.

Keep learning

Digital technology and online gaming provide many opportunities for learning and increasing knowledge. Research in the past five years has started to document some of the benefits experienced by children and adolescents. According to Isabela Granic, a researcher at Radboud University Nijmegen in the Netherlands, many video games provide young people with social, cognitive, and emotional experiences and can also boost wellbeing.[22] Social games allow children and young people to test out different life scenarios, which provide great opportunities to develop skills that will be helpful in similar, real-life scenarios. There are also well-documented cognitive benefits, including creativity, spatial reasoning, logical thinking, and teamwork. Video games can give young people a temporary escape from a negative life situation like bullying and allow them to experience moments of pride, achievement, and a sense of mastery.

For some young people, gaming might provide an opportunity to feel capable in a way that they don't in the non-digital world. Often the characters they adopt are athletic and highly skilled in their accomplishments. The immediate feedback from their performance can also be helpful for young people who might feel they don't get this in the non-digital world, and this can make the gaming experience even more important to a child.

Why is it so hard to get my child off their screen?

As a parent, trying to encourage my child to get off their screen, or not think about it, is often painful and sometimes explosive. There are several reasons why young people get so hooked on video gaming and other forms of digital media.

Dopamine
Russell Poldrack, professor of psychology at Stanford University, calls dopamine the "gimme more" neurotransmitter, because once we have experienced a hit of dopamine, our brains automatically crave more.[23]

As described above, dopamine not only activates desire (for the attractive person across the room, the delicious cake in the window, the designer trainers that someone we admire wears), it also gives us the energy, focus and tenacity to get the thing that is the object of our desire. It supports us to plan and strategize as to how we might do that best, giving us a sense of reward when we achieve the goal. Dopamine likes new things, unexpected wins; the thrill of the chase. It's less interested in the here and now and enjoying the moment. So, when we get to our goal, if something new or better comes along, it will sweep us right back up with the chase again. It wants to keep us moving, exploring, dreaming, wanting more. Even better, if you can do this with others in a team, with a shared goal. Sound familiar?

It's no coincidence that dopamine and video gaming go together like birds of a feather. In 2022, across-the-world revenue from video gaming was $184.4 billion. Similarly, digital entertainment and social media create billions in revenue. Behind these figures lie huge levels of investment and expertise in making sure we keep coming back for more, along with all the data that informs what's most effective at keeping us engaged. So, it makes sense that the programmers behind these games and platforms will have found the most effective ways to hijack our dopamine systems and keep us chasing the dream and wanting more. It also makes sense that policymakers need to ensure these companies act responsibly and help protect young people's mental health—not exploit it.

Novelty bias

Our brains have something that researchers call a novelty bias, which means they are built to seek out and attend to anything new that is happening in our environment. Computer games (and screens in general) present a constantly changing environment, which is specifically designed to hold our attention and, unlike with other activities, which have a natural ending, many of the current games have no ending cues. This means that they are essentially a bottomless pit of novelty capturing and holding attention: "I can't stop the game, Mom, I'll die!"

Withdrawal and craving more

Although research is still unclear, mounting evidence suggests that video games do not lead to a significant increase in aggression in the long term. However, we will all have experienced moments when our young person will resist coming off a screen and may get aggressive when we insist they do.

Throughout the day we transition from one activity to another and, for the most part, we don't even notice because it happens automatically. Young people, particularly those with neurodiversity (like autism or ADHD), may find these transitions difficult, as it involves change and a shift in attention. Making a transition from something totally absorbing back to reality can be especially difficult and sometimes lead to conflict. Understanding brain chemistry can help make sense of this reaction.

The dopamine crash

As the screen-based activity is feeding their brain with the rewarding feelings that come from dopamine, immediately following coming off the screen, our child can experience a brief period of withdrawal (a bit like someone taking away a delicious bowl of ice cream when you're halfway through). I like to understand it as the brain needing to recalibrate without the stimulation of the game ("Hey, give me that back! I want to keep eating that ice cream!"). During this recalibration (which might only be a matter of minutes), the brain experiences a dopamine crash as the stimulation is taken away—making you feel terrible, craving that thing, wanting it back to take away the pain of the crash. However, the brain needs to experience this crash to be able to return to normal levels of dopamine production and get back on track and on with the day, without the stimulant in question (game or ice cream).

Fight-flight

Some video games, particularly those with a focus on survival, can activate what we call the fight-flight (stress) response in the brain (see chapter 7). When this happens, our bodies are flooded with the stress neurochemicals adrenaline and cortisol. These increase our heart rate and make us more aware of and responsive to danger, which can improve strength and focus. This focus can help pursue a target with more precision. While fight-flight is activated, your child is likely to become more frustrated and angry (with themselves or others), and in this heightened state of arousal, you may see them getting distressed in their game and also struggle to transition calmly away from their device.

Essentially, the powerful effect screens have on our children's and teenagers' brains and bodies means they need special handling as they disengage from the exciting worlds in which they've been fully immersed. They also benefit from being taught about this process, so they can be more aware of how they might need your support until they get better at self-managing these addictive elements.

Top tips for managing the highs and lows of gaming and screen time

▶ Avoid turning your child's game off without warning. A bit like getting something you're enjoying unexpectedly removed—you're going to get a reaction.

▶ Create as much predictability as possible about screen time coming to an end and have a clear plan with the young person about a place in the game/activity they can safely get to before the screen is turned off (e.g., "We're going to eat at 6:30 p.m. today, so please can you start to finish your playing time at 6:00 p.m.? I can remind you when there's five minutes to go, if you would like me to").

▶ Try not to be reactive during the dopamine-crash phase, as this is when things tend to escalate, which can increase the probability of more distress and anger. I avoid giving my kids a lecture, or pointing out why I don't like them playing on the game, as this leads to further conflict.

- ▸ Explain to your children, when they are calm, about the dopamine crash and how they can expect to feel unhappy and angry as they come off their device. Help them understand that this feeling will pass, and work out together how you can limit the damage during this transition. Agree together on things that might help (e.g., a five-minute warning, not shouting, moving to another room away from the device). This will help these blips not get undue attention or ruin the day.

- ▸ Some children/teenagers may find certain games too stimulating or triggering of the fight-flight response, leading to high levels of frustration while playing and more difficulties when they come off the game. These same children may find they can enjoy other games which are less adrenaline-inducing, without these fallouts (e.g., Minecraft, Roblox). Depending on the age of your child and the level of the fallout, you might have to restrict some games until they are more able to cope with the demands of the game in question.

- ▸ Create routines and structures that protect certain times from gaming/devices (e.g., times when devices are off for the whole family, like mealtimes; times when the Wi-Fi is off to enable other ways of interacting). Introducing these changes can create an initial negative reaction, but children quickly adjust if these rules are explained to them, are fair, and are consistent—and you follow them, too.

- ▸ Ensuring access to a range of learning experiences, not just those experienced on devices, is important to allow them to develop a balanced approach to engaging with learning and activities. Providing access to alternative activities—even if they are linked to those games of interest (e.g., playing football in the garden, as well as playing football online, learning to draw manga characters as well as playing or watching anime, building Lego worlds as well as playing Lego Batman). You can make these in-person activities more appealing by getting involved or showing an interest in the end product (the model or picture). Even just watching your child kick a football around will bring them joy.

> ▶ Provide opportunities for a sense of mastery outside of gaming to encourage your child to feel that gaming is not the only place they experience this feeling. Supporting our children to feel good about things they can make and do—whether that is cooking, sports, building things, telling stories, creating things with art or other materials, or making music—can ensure our children are not just getting their sense of learning and achievement by putting effort in online, but also through other activities that activate dopamine and other neurochemicals that help them enjoy the here and now. You may need to invest some time in supporting them to become more skilled at these activities. Just remember, providing your input "little and often" is more helpful than intense input irregularly.

Flow

Have you ever been so involved in an enjoyable activity that nothing else seemed to matter? A task that felt challenging, but achievable, too? Where your actions and awareness were merged and you no longer felt self-conscious or caught up in rumination?

If so, this is probably what psychologist Mihaly Csikszentmihalyi describes as "Flow."[24] Csikszentmihalyi found that people who had the experience of becoming completely absorbed in an activity that was challenging enough to stretch them, but not so difficult as to frustrate them or to be unachievable, had higher levels of contentment. Researchers have also since found people get more pleasure out of flow activities when doing them with others.

Sometimes the digital world can create opportunities for our children to experience flow—a game where their skills are perfectly matched to the task, and they are not over-activated (frustrated or distressed; e.g., a high-adrenaline adventure game) or under-activated (bored or passive; e.g., watching a TV show or scrolling through social media). An example of a flow activity might be a child lost in the experience of creating a Minecraft world.

Distraction destroys flow, so a busy environment with lots of distractions reduces this opportunity. Providing opportunities for our children to engage in flow activities beyond the digital world can encourage these positive experiences that activate the much-needed here-and-now neurochemicals, which are good for brain development and wellbeing. Activities that involve movement (sports, dance) and creative activities (drawing, building, playing an instrument, writing, reading, cooking) are particularly good at encouraging this. The key to flow is doing something you enjoy where the challenge and skill are matched.

ACTIVITY BOX

Write down activities your child does that encourage flow. Which of these activities do not involve digital devices? What activities do you do that encourage flow? How could you encourage more opportunities for flow in your and your child's day? Remember: five to ten minutes is enough.

Be giving

As a single parent working full-time, I'm hugely reliant on screens to keep my children occupied and to reduce conflict in my household. If each of my children is busy in their own virtual world, they don't seem to aggravate each other, make a mess, or be itching to get out and do something I won't have oversight of. Typically, while they are busy on their devices, I'm busy on mine. This has huge value to me. I find myself feeling guilty about this and worrying that I've failed as a parent.

Young people are astute observers of the world around them. It's now well established that they are much more influenced by what we do, as opposed to what we say. My children constantly remind me when I ask them to come off their screen that I'm always on mine, and that I don't listen to them when I am. My excuse is, "Yes, but I'm working," or, "I need to check grandma is OK." In some ways, my excuses are not much different from theirs. This is a work-in-progress for me: giving my time to my children, with the use of screens or not.

The biggest win for me as an exhausted mom at the end of the day is to sit with my son or daughter and watch a program together we're both into. (I've managed to watch *Stranger Things* with each of my three children!) We both look forward to these moments of being together and sharing a screen-based story. When I'm away from my children, I try to give them my attention by sending an encouraging text message or a photo—showing I'm holding them in mind. This is especially important as they live away from me part of the time with their dad. If I have more energy, joining them (with their permission) in their online world can be helpful, perhaps making time to create a TikTok video or play a game together. This has the double benefit of increasing my understanding of why this activity is so attractive, while also allowing me to give more quality time to my children, on their terms, in their expert area.

Digital technology provides the opportunity to give our positive energy to others. It also offers many opportunities to take away our time and energy. It's a constant battle for me to find the balance. To consciously use the technology to help give myself and others positive time and energy, and not get drawn into draining my time and energy with things that feel unproductive and unkind. In theory, digital technology should increase our time for other activities if we use it consciously and wisely.

Finding balance

Screen time and the use of digital technology are complicated subjects. There are no set answers. Black-and-white recommendations can be comforting when we feel out of our depth, so this lack of clarity may feel frustrating. I've tried to liberate myself from rules and instead ask this key question to help me on a daily basis: is the way my family and I are using digital technology helping or hindering me in the areas of the Wellbeing Abacus? What small things can I do more of, which increase the positive influence and protect against the negative? I also consider what other things might be happening in my child's life which may impact them emotionally and may lead them to disproportionately rely on their screens.

Knowing I'm competing with a multibillion-dollar industry means I give my children and myself less of a hard time when they resist coming off their screens. It's not my fault or theirs that a day on the beach doesn't offer the same excitement it might have done for me as a child. But they still come off their gadgets, and we still go to the beach. I hold onto the belief that spending authentic time together with my children, my friends and family is most valuable to myself and them—this could be with the help of digital technology or not.

There are well-evidenced apps that provide information and support to young people struggling with low mood, anxiety, and other difficulties (find some on page 308). Signposting our children to these resources so they are close at hand in a medium they can access easily could be helpful for them.

The future

Digital technology will continue to grow and develop and become more sophisticated and ingrained in our lives. Our children are likely to quickly become more skilled and savvier than us in this area! They are not only the current users of technology; they are also the future programmers and creators in this area. They may become the policy-makers who can influence how this powerful medium is regulated. We may have to use their experience to teach us, and our younger children, about how to manage this world.

Although there are many structural ways we can support our young people to manage their time and the content they are exposed to on their devices, such as ensuring computers are turned off after certain times in the evening and using parental controls, ultimately our leverage with our young person is our relationship with them. By helping them to understand both the positives and negatives of technology and taking the time to actively listen to their concerns, we will be in a much better position to find a balance together in a supportive and collaborative way. Head to the resource pack for additional resources to support you in this quest.

ACTIVITY BOX

Look at the table below. What small changes can you make in each area of wellbeing to encourage balance in the use of digital technology in your family? I have shared the things I am working on.

Connect with others	Privileging in-person opportunities even if it is more hassle
Physical activity	Use app to track activity
Sleep	Build relaxation app into bedtime routine
Nutrition	Phones/screens away at mealtimes
Take notice	Not look at my phone when walking around; instead, look up at the world
Keep learning	Take a non-judgmental interest in what my children are learning online
Be giving	Give encouragement to friends/family through messaging

SUMMARY

→ Digital technology is woven into the fabric of our lives. We can't ignore its impact on family life.

→ The research is unclear about its impact on mental health. The focus should be less on how much time we spend on screens and more on what we do on them.

→   We can use screens to either facilitate or disrupt each of the seven areas of wellbeing:

- Social connection can be supported with digital technology. It can also be disrupted by negative interactions and preoccupations with popularity. Supporting our children with curiosity and opportunities to make sense of these interactions will help protect them from the negative elements.

- The relationship between sleep, physical activity, eating behaviors, and excessive screen time use is complicated. Making small, practical changes and having insight into what's going on in our child's emotional world can help protect against difficulties in this area.

- Digital technology provides many opportunities for learning and a sense of mastery. Gaming and social media are designed to be as attractive as possible to encourage their continued use. It can therefore be hard to control how much time we spend on them. Providing boundaries around this and access to other non-digital activities can help our children build balance in this area.

- Digital technology can distract us from enjoying the moment and taking notice of the world around us. Providing opportunities for "flow" activities can encourage wellbeing.

- Using technology to help us spend more time with our children and important others can be surprisingly difficult. However, small changes in our approach can make a big difference.

→   Our relationship with our children is pivotal in helping us simultaneously protect and encourage them to safely explore the digital world—a world they will inevitably influence as adults.

PART 2
Difficult Feelings

The good, the bad, and the ugly

Chapter 4

The link between feelings and behavior

There is nothing better than those joyful times when we experience the pleasure of love and belonging. Holding a lover's hand at a gig, messing around with a best friend on a summer's day, gazing in wonder at your newborn baby—all invoke such feelings. But these glorious moments cannot last forever.

It's likely you're reading this book because less-welcome feelings are showing up in your family and causing problems: anger, sadness, anxiety, grief, fear, loneliness. These emotions can trigger distress and take over in ways that create internal and external conflict. As parents, we may be frustrated by our children sometimes being unable to regulate their emotions, such as explosive anger that leads to destructive actions and defiance. Other times, we might not be able to understand emotions our children are feeling or why, leaving us feeling confused and worried. We may see our children caught in intense angst and feel them withdrawing from us, and even engaging in harmful behaviors in an attempt to cope.

Successfully managing emotions is vital for positive mental health, good social relationships and academic achievement. As our children develop, learning how to deal with their feelings is one of the most important tasks they will face. As they grow up, they may experience extreme emotions in response to the things that happen to them. Our task as parents or carers is to help our children make sense of these feelings and learn how to use them helpfully. This process is called emotional regulation. It also involves teaching them the consequences of behaviors that overstep the mark. This is not always easy—especially when we throw our own emotions into the mix.

This section of the book explores why feelings are so important, the neuroscience behind emotions, and how we as parents can practically support our children to develop good emotional regulation.

Do I need to worry about my child?

Difficulties with mental health and relationships tend to emerge when young people:

* struggle to understand and communicate their feelings effectively; and/or
* those around them do not provide them with the support they need.

This means their emotional needs are not met. It can lead to behaviors that are challenging, as well as feelings of anxiety, low mood, and self-harm.

In my experience, most young people I see are struggling with their mental health because they are overwhelmed by feelings they don't want or understand. I help them make sense of these emotions in the context of the things that are happening in their lives. The majority of adolescents I work with usually tell me they've tried various ways to cope with difficult feelings. Often, they attempt to push them deeper inside, but they then find that these feelings come back even stronger than before. Many try to find ways to manage them; perhaps through controlling their thoughts (obsessive thinking patterns), what they eat (eating disorders), or physical pain (self-harm). Often the adults around them see a very different version of what's going on inside them, such as perceiving them as a defiant or withdrawn child, rather than a young person in emotional distress. This often leaves the young person feeling misunderstood and alone.

Sometimes, younger children are referred to me because they seem to have lost control of their emotions to the point that they are not able to conform to the expected home and school rules without huge outbursts, sometimes to the point they are hurting themselves or others.

Although these are perhaps the more extreme examples, the simple truth is, for all of us, life throws up difficulties that will lead to strong emotions. These in turn will influence what happens next (what we do), our relationships with others and the world, and how we feel about ourselves.

It's natural that as our children experience hardship and difficulties, they will need help from those around them to understand what they are feeling and why, and to learn to communicate their needs to others. If we can support our children to build skills in this area, we support their wellbeing, as well as their ability to learn and build positive relationships.

Young people who may need more support in this area tend to:

* be sensitive to being triggered more quickly by events, both internal (e.g., self-criticism) and external (e.g., being told off)—which brings about strong feelings quickly (others feel they have to walk on eggshells to avoid outbursts);

* take a long time to settle down once they've been distressed;

* experience emotions more intensely and seem to have a disproportionate response to a situation.

Children who struggle in this way will especially benefit from the tools in this section of the book. As emotions are a fundamental part of being human, these tools apply to all children and adults and are effective in building good emotional regulation for everyone. If you're interested in some of the reasons why children might struggle more in these areas, take a look at "Trauma: What happened to us?" in chapter 5.

Why emotions are important

Emotions ensure we evolve and survive. They do this through helping us:

* identify and respond quickly to threats (protection);
* motivate and develop ourselves (motivation);
* communicate with those around us (connection); and
* make life worth living (enjoyment).

This process creates changes both **physically** (e.g., an increase in heart rate) and **psychologically** (our thoughts and feelings) and hugely impacts our behavior.

Emotions tend to be triggered by external events and internal thoughts. Essentially, they are a messaging system letting us know how things are going in our world and propelling us to take action. Influenced by our past experiences, they are often multilayered and complicated. Rarely do we experience one emotion in isolation. Being able to identify and communicate them appropriately is critical in improving self-awareness, building meaningful connections with others, and making good decisions.

What emotions might look like in a child

As we mature into adulthood, we learn to use language to express our emotions and hide some of the physical cues that show we're distressed (I feel like screaming, but instead I explain, "I'm frustrated") or excited (I feel like jumping for joy, but say, "That's great news"). As younger children are less able to communicate their feelings with words, the clues to their emotions are often in what they do with their bodies (their behavior). To help make the link between your child's behavior and their feelings, look at the activity below to explore how your child might communicate their feelings through their behaviors, and see if these behaviors are helpful in getting their emotional needs met.

ACTIVITY BOX

In the table below, you'll see a range of emotions that your child might experience, and how these might present as behaviors. I have completed the table with an example scenario. On your own piece of paper: (1) Write down a situation where you might see your child in distress; (2) Write down the behaviors you see in your child in this situation; (3) Write down any emotions they might be a sign of; (4) Lastly, write down the response your child might get from others based on this behavior.

1. Situation	Sister stole sweets
2. External behavior	Shouting, crying, throwing/hitting, saying cruel things, running away, impulsive/more energy, refusing to communicate, unable to talk, physically hurting self, withdrawing from others, becoming more controlling, black-and-white thinking
3. Internal emotion	**Anger,** sadness, fear, shame, guilt, envy, jealousy, disgust, interest, surprise, joy
4. Response from others	Using a loud, angry voice to enforce sanctions (e.g., "You are going to have to go to your room for 10 minutes now and no more X-Box!")

Sometimes, emotions trigger behaviors that help get the response from others required to meet emotional needs (e.g., when my son's pet died, he cried. I responded with comforting words and a cuddle). Other times, emotions trigger behaviors that get a response from others that does not get emotional needs met (e.g., when my son was angry because his sister took his sweets, he hit her. I responded with shouting and sanctions for him, which led to increased feelings of being treated unfairly and anger in my son). Look back at your example above; did your child's behavior lead to their emotional need being met?

Choose one of your child's external behaviors that you find most tricky. What might be the underlying emotion? How helpful, or unhelpful, is this behavior in getting their underlying emotional need(s) met?

How big feelings take over

Every parent knows that big feelings can take over during emotion-filled moments. They can hijack the family when another member is experiencing them. As important as feelings are in helping us live a full and meaningful life, they can sometimes get in the way of learning and maintaining positive relationships.

Most families and young people I work with are struggling in one way or another with strong emotions. These feelings might make them explode, shut down, become uncooperative or destructive (e.g., anger, fear). There are some emotions that they might try to push away (e.g., sadness, shame), but which keep coming back. To help families understand these issues, I find explaining how the brain works in simple terms can make sense of what's happening inside a young person in these moments of distress. This new knowledge takes away some of the frustration and guilt that is felt by not being able to manage these feelings. At this point I can share the tools that will help in these situations, and family members understand why they work.

The Brain House

Clinical professor of psychiatry Dr. Dan Siegel and pediatric and adolescent psychotherapist Dr. Tina Payne Bryson talk about the brain being like a house,[25] an analogy I often explain to families. We can think of this as a brain being split into two, with an upstairs and a downstairs.

The downstairs brain

The downstairs (emotional limbic) brain is where our emotions live: anger, happiness, fear, and excitement. It's also the alarm system in our brain, detecting when things are unsafe. All about survival, it's constantly keeping an eye out for things (fight-flight, chapter 7) and making sure we get out of danger quickly. When we're born, this part of the brain is well developed and works automatically. It's what makes babies cry when they are hungry, cold or scared. Closely linked to the body's physiological system (autonomic nervous system), it sends bodily signals, which act as an effective way of communicating (crying, smiling, writhing limbs, arms that reach out). It tells us as parents to look after our baby (feed them, keep them warm, dry and clean) and make sure they stay out of danger. As a baby matures into a child, this is the system they will rely on to get themselves out of danger (e.g., running, fighting, freezing).

The upstairs brain

The upstairs (thinking–prefrontal cortex) brain is the control tower of our brain, where language develops, as well as our ability to organize ourselves, problem-solve and describe how we're feeling. It helps us think about things logically. The upstairs part of our brain is not devel-

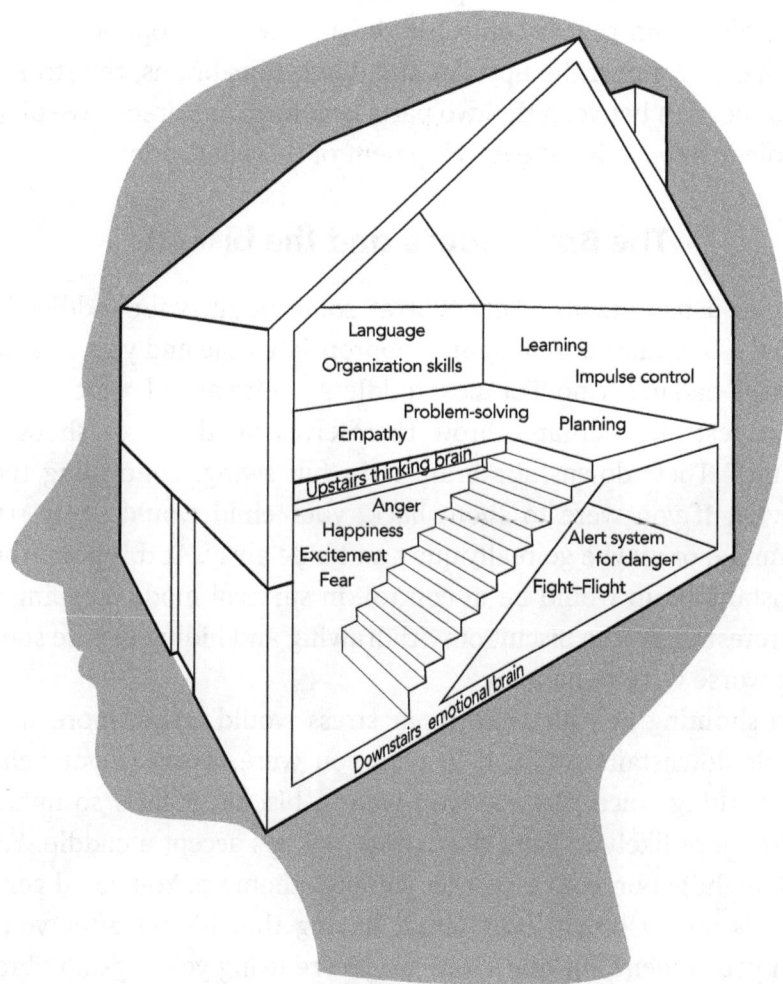

Language
Organization skills
Learning
Impulse control
Problem-solving
Planning
Empathy
Upstairs thinking brain
Anger
Happiness
Excitement
Fear
Alert system
for danger
Fight–Flight
Downstairs emotional brain

oped when we're born, and it takes around twenty-four years for this part of the brain to fully do so. As our children grow, we need to provide them with learning experiences that will help develop this area of the brain.

The staircase

As you can see in the diagram (p. 87), there is a staircase between the upstairs and downstairs brain. This connection is what helps the downstairs brain communicate with the upstairs brain and make sense of what to do in any situation. If the downstairs brain is getting over-excited or upset, the upstairs brain can help work out what's needed to resolve the problem, take planned action and then signal to the downstairs brain that it can settle down. The more opportunities a child has to connect the upstairs and downstairs brains, the stronger the connection between the two parts becomes. As parents, we play a key role in supporting the development of this connection.

The Brain House and the biscuit

If you're a parent, it's likely that at some point, your toddler has wanted a biscuit or a treat at an inappropriate time and you, as a parent, have had to say no. For most toddlers, their natural response is to cry, protest and perhaps throw themselves on the floor shouting, "Biscuit!" Their downstairs brain is in full swing, controlling their behavior. If you were to shout back, your child would likely start screaming, or maybe go really quiet and hide away. At this point their downstairs brain would be in control, in survival mode, keeping up the protest to get the biscuit or withdrawing and hiding in case something worse were to happen.

In shouting at your child, your stress would create more stress in their downstairs brain. If instead you were to say to your child in a soothing voice, "I know you want a biscuit, it feels so unfair," they're more likely to calm down and perhaps accept a cuddle. Your child might get on your lap or let you pick them up. You could gently say, "It's nearly lunch; how about having that biscuit after you've eaten your lunch?" In that moment, you're using your upstairs brain to connect with your child's downstairs brain, reassuring them by making them feel safe again: "It's OK, you can calm down. Nothing bad is going to happen. You can get your biscuit later." You have loaned your child your upstairs brain to help them regulate their own emotions. Even if they might not like the outcome, with your help they've been able to tolerate this feeling. The more opportunities your child has to experience their downstairs brain being soothed by their own or your upstairs brain, the stronger the connection grows between the two and the better they get at regulating their emotions.

Think of a time when you have loaned your child your upstairs brain to help reduce their distress. Start noticing when you do this effectively. It will help give clues as to what works well with your child (e.g., speaking in a calm voice, taking a pause before reacting, giving your child space when they are upset). See chapter 5 for top tips on how to do this.

Flipping the lid

You might have personally experienced or witnessed, in your child and other adults, the downstairs brain hijacking the upstairs brain. Drs. Dan Siegel and Tina Payne Bryson use the term "flipping the lid" to describe this. If you look at the illustration on page 91, you can see that as the downstairs brain gets more activated, the upstairs brain literally "flips off" the downstairs brain, like the lid of a box. When this happens, we can't listen to others or to logic—it all becomes white noise as our logical thinking brains are disconnected. This is our brain's way of protecting us from danger. After all, the downstairs brain likes to be in control to ensure it's doing the most important job of all—looking after us. It acts quickly because it knows in a dangerous situation it needs to. It doesn't want to be slowed down by the upstairs brain, so it literally cuts the connection to protect us. However, in taking over, this can sometimes make us behave in ways that unhelpfully add to distress. For many young people this might be shouting, crying, hitting out, running away or, for some of our adolescents, we may see them storm off, slam doors and isolate themselves where they might in their distress hurt themselves.

ACTIVITY BOX

Think of a recent scenario when your child has "flipped their lid" and write it down before answering these questions.

1. How did you know your child had flipped their lid (e.g., screaming, crying, hitting, running away, withdrawing)?

2. What had happened just before?

3. What emotions/feelings do you think your child was experiencing?

4. How did others around your child respond?

5. Did this response help, or make the situation worse?

6. Did your child have a better understanding of themselves at the end of this event?

7. If your child was less driven by the downstairs brain, what might they have been able to do differently?

Chapter 5 covers how to respond if your child is flipping their lid.

Fact Box

Brain changes in adolescence

From the ages of thirteen to twenty-four, a lot of change occurs in both the upstairs and downstairs brain (we will discuss this more in chapter 14). During adolescence, the downstairs brain can become more sensitive to threat cues, especially anything related to things not going well socially. The upstairs brain is also busy reorganizing itself, preparing for adulthood. This means adolescence is a tricky time for managing strong feelings, especially if the staircase is not as strong as it could be.

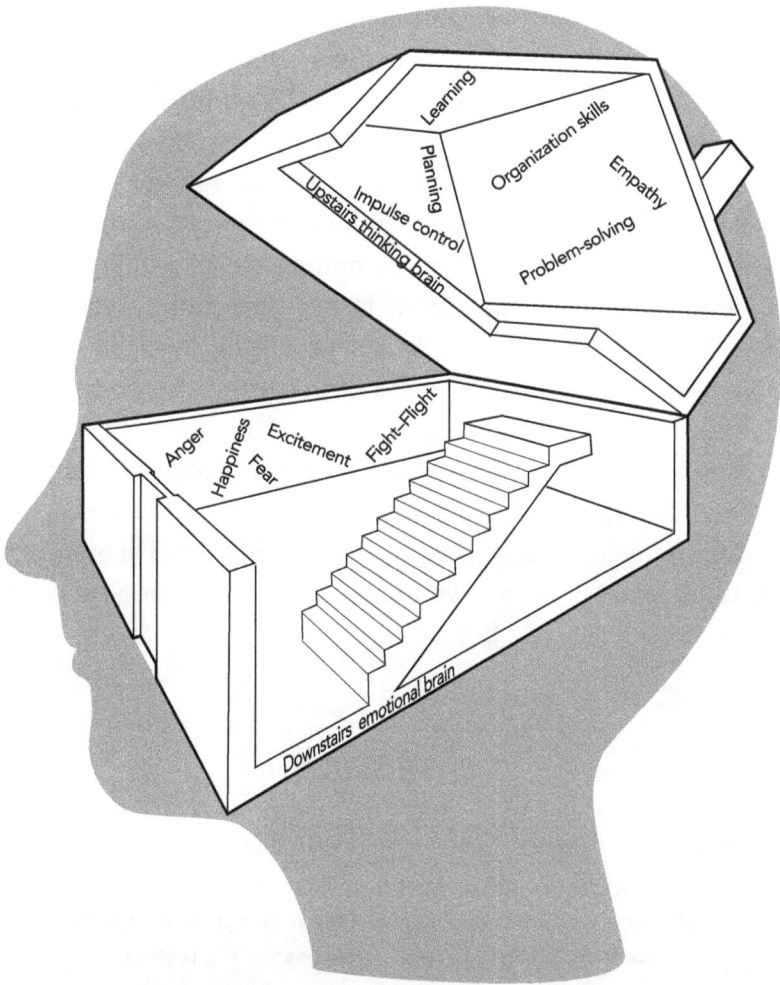

Learning

Planning

Organization skills

Empathy

Impulse control

Upstairs thinking brain

Problem-solving

Anger   Happiness   Excitement   Fight-Flight

Fear

Downstairs emotional brain

When you flip your lid

Flipping lids can be contagious in families in high-stress situations. In many families, the increase in stress can lead to other family members flipping their lids (both siblings and parents). Our children often know how to press our buttons. Their behavior can be a trigger for us feeling overwhelmed when dealing with the daily challenges of parenthood and life.

Personally, one of my biggest challenges is trying not to overreact when one of my children has been rude or aggressive to me or their siblings in the throes of flipping their lid. This is further compounded if I'm feeling tired after a long day. When I flip my lid and say unhelpful things, it creates more emotional distress for me and my child, and impacts our relationship. It's a difficult cycle from which to break free.

This may be a familiar scene to many parents reading this page. We will all have our own versions in our households, and will have experienced our own versions in our families growing up. This is a natural reflection of the challenges of living together with those we love, while navigating the demands of life and relationships. This part of the book is all about offering you insight into how and why we get into these unhelpful scenarios and giving you the tools to approach them differently to increase integration, flexibility and adaptability for a better outcome for you and your family. Let's have a look at what this looks like in Bella's story, below.

- -

CASE STUDY

Bella's Story (Part 1)

We will follow Bella and her parents through the next two chapters as they try out some of the tools I'm sharing with you to help manage and make sense of big feelings.

The problem
Meet the Johnsons. Bella is twelve years old, and both her mom and stepdad need support. Bella has been struggling with big outbursts of destructive behavior. She can hit out, or break things and the family is worried about her hurting herself and her younger sibling when she's in a rage.

The family situation
Bella lived most of the week with her dad until she was ten, but for the last two years has been living most of the week with her mom, stepdad, and baby

half-brother. Bella explained that life at her mom's was settled and predictable, with lots of good routines and warm care. She described that things at her dad's house were less predictable, with fewer rules and routines.

When things get difficult
To understand things better, I asked Bella's mom and stepdad about the time or situation when things were most tricky for Bella. They explained that Bella spent some weekends with Dad, and it was when she came home from staying at her dad's house that things would get most difficult. Bella would be grumpy, but say she was fine when asked what was wrong. The smallest thing would upset her and, from there, things would escalate to the point that everyone in the house would become upset and scared.

The Brain House
To help make sense of what might be going on for Bella, I introduced the Johnsons to the Brain House. We looked at a Sunday evening when Bella got home from her dad's and her behavior got difficult to map what was happening to the brains in the household. We worked out that Bella's downstairs brain was very sensitive when she returned from her dad's as she had lots of emotions swirling around. Mom would then ask Bella to do something like come off her computer for dinner and Bella would flip her lid, shouting and refusing.

The flip-the-lid cycle
Mom would then flip her lid and turn the computer off. Bella's fight-flight downstairs brain would then take over and she might throw the remote and break something or run to her bedroom to escape the situation. Bella's mom would then get more cross in her "flipped-lid" place, and follow her around, often with a raised voice. Bella said being told the consequences for her behavior and Mom following her around telling her off was keeping her downstairs brain in full meltdown mode. They both understood that their flipped lids were staying flipped and leading to behaviors they both regretted afterwards. Mom could see that her flipped-lid reaction was contributing to Bella's distress and not helping her daughter get her upstairs brain reconnected to her downstairs brain (see the illustration on page 94).

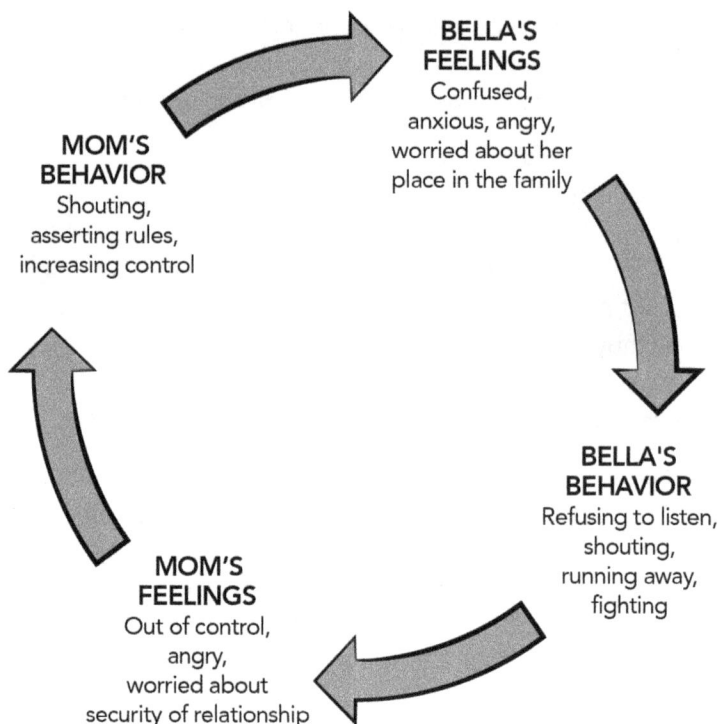

BELLA'S FEELINGS
Confused, anxious, angry, worried about her place in the family

MOM'S BEHAVIOR
Shouting, asserting rules, increasing control

BELLA'S BEHAVIOR
Refusing to listen, shouting, running away, fighting

MOM'S FEELINGS
Out of control, angry, worried about security of relationship

The flip-the-lid triggers

In this discussion, Bella's parents were able to understand that her difficult behaviors did not come out of the blue. They were triggered by the big feelings she was having transitioning from one household to another. Bella's mom was able to recognize that her response to Bella's behavior was based on her "feeling out of control of Bella and worrying she doesn't want to live with me," triggering her to flip her lid. Although in the moment, she felt like she was doing the right thing in her role as a parent to try to stop the destructive behaviors and be sure Bella understood their consequences, she saw how she was unintentionally contributing to the difficult cycle.

Breaking the cycle

This new insight into the family's worst night of the week helped demystify Bella's behavior and reduce blame. It also helped us think together how we could change the situation or people's behavior to support getting the upstairs brain reconnected with the downstairs brain to break the flipped-lid cycle. See how we do this with the Johnsons in the next chapter.

In the resource pack you will find a flip-the-lid cycle worksheet that you can complete for you and your child. Consider what triggers are particularly challenging for your child and what triggers are particularly challenging for you.

Balancing emotions with learning the rules of life

In the case example above, Bella and her mom's flip-the-lid cycle reflects the tension we face as parents between keeping our children safe and teaching them acceptable behaviors, while supporting their emotional development. Without this guidance, children will struggle to function well in their family and in other social situations (e.g., school, going to friends' homes, playing sports). In the scenario where my son hit his sister when she stole his sweets, if he doesn't learn to manage his anger without hitting others, and learn that this behavior is socially unacceptable, it will have an impact on his ability to learn and build positive relationships. Sometimes a child will flip their lid in response to us or another adult asking them to do something they do not want to do. They will need to learn to do the things they don't like—you can't avoid every difficult situation. We can't not ask them to do the things they need to do because of fear of them flipping their lid.

Bella's mom's response to Bella's distressed behavior and her unwillingness to do what she asked was because she wanted to ensure Bella didn't hurt herself or anyone else and understood her behavior was unacceptable. This is an essential and sometimes difficult part of being a good parent. Bella's mom's reaction to her behavior was out of love, because she cares about Bella and wants her to grow into a well-rounded individual who feels happy about her life and respects societal rules. Unfortunately, because Bella was in distress and her upstairs brain was disconnected from her downstairs brain, she was not able to experience Mom's input as helpful guidance she could learn from. Instead, it was experienced as another threat or overwhelming. When our children are in distress, or emotional pain, they cannot learn, as the upstairs brain is disconnected and not tuned into the world around them.

This is where understanding the Brain House provides the key to helping us as parents to successfully do both caring and teaching the rules of life. For Bella's family, the Brain House helped them understand that when Bella was experiencing strong feelings, her brain had a biological reaction, sending her into fight-flight mode and switching off her ability to listen to others and be cooperative. In those moments, Bella's parents' response unintentionally contributed to her staying in fight-flight mode. But importantly, as they had Bella's best interests at heart, they wanted to understand how to find another way to show her they cared, while also providing clear boundaries.

The Brain House demonstrates that in these scenarios our biggest chance of success in communicating effectively with our child is to support them to reconnect their upstairs and downstairs brain— *before* we go on to provide them with the necessary guidance to correct their behavior.

I'm sure as you finish reading this chapter you're asking, as the Johnsons did: how do we teach our children to respect familial and societal rules, while also helping them to feel their emotions and communicate without sabotaging themselves and/or their relationships with others? How do those of us with busy and demanding lives, with likely more than one child, achieve this?

In the next two chapters, I'll outline the key tools that will enable you as parents to quickly support your child and reconnect their downstairs and upstairs brain so your child can effectively learn:

1. the rules of life through collaboration and shared problem-solving;

2. how to tune into difficult feelings so they can see how these feelings are signposts to what's important to them, rather than something they need to escape;

3. how to use their feelings to make good decisions about what to do next.

These simple tools are easy to do for a few seconds a day, and enough to build strong emotional regulation, and help your family become a calmer, more positive place to be.

ACTIVITY BOX

Sharing the Brain House with your child is really helpful in creating a shared language in your family to aid increased awareness of how they are feeling and what their brain might be doing in high-stress moments.

With this tool, your child will get better at noticing what's going on for them ("I need to take some time out or I'll flip my lid") and for others ("I think Mom is about to flip her lid. I'd better not press her buttons!"). Show your child the picture of the Brain House on page 87—explain about the downstairs and upstairs brain. Younger children may enjoy drawing their own picture and creating characters that live in the downstairs brain (Mr. Angry, Miss Happy, Dr. "Keep Safe") and upstairs brain (Ms. Organized, Mrs. Logical, Mr. Problem Solving). They may identify that some characters are bossier than others, which can sometimes be helpful and sometimes not. Think together about what helps the two floors stay connected to develop practical ideas you can use to support them.

SUMMARY

→ Difficulties with mental health and relationships tend to emerge when young people struggle to understand and communicate their feelings effectively.

→ Big feelings are often communicated through behavior; sometimes this behavior is challenging and leads to further emotional distress in families.

→   To support healthy emotional development in our child, it's important to understand what happens to the brain when we experience strong emotions. The Brain House is a helpful way to do this.

→   We have a downstairs brain, which is our alert system for danger. It gives us our fight-flight response and is where our feelings/ emotions live.

→   We have an upstairs brain, which is our control tower. It's where logical thinking takes place and helps us to organize ourselves, communicate through language, make decisions, and learn.

→   The connection between the upstairs and downstairs brain is like a staircase that helps our child feel important feelings and do what they need to in response to them to both stay safe and lead a good life.

→   When experiencing emotional distress, the upstairs brain becomes disconnected from the downstairs brain ("flip the lid"). When this happens, it's difficult to be cooperative or learn because the upstairs brain is "offline." Unintentionally, as parents we can contribute to the flip-the-lid cycle, leading to increased distress in our child. Becoming more aware of the flip-the-lid cycle can help us break free from it.

→   All children need help from the adults around them to: (a) regulate their emotions (build a strong connection—the staircase—between the upstairs and downstairs brain), and (b) learn how to use their feelings to make good decisions. How to do this successfully is covered in the next two chapters.

Chapter 5

Connection before correction

Recently, I crashed my car on my way to a holiday at my mom's. It was a stressful experience, but, despite being stuck in the central reservation of the motorway with my three kids on a Friday night at rush hour, I felt grateful that we were not hurt, aware that we were in physical danger and totally dependent on the many strangers required to help me and my kids out of this dangerous situation. When we were picked up by the rescue truck two hours later, we were literally elated. The sense of safety and relief we felt knowing we were OK was incredible. We told everyone we knew what had happened and shared photos; their reactions reinforced our sense of luckiness and helped us understand the experience. The story became reframed as an adventure rather than a traumatic event. Our feelings of stress and fear became those of relief.

Eight weeks later, a brown envelope arrived in the post. I opened it and was shocked to see "Civil Court Order" for a lot of money from a name I did not recognize. In that moment, I was flooded with shock, incomprehension and, most overwhelmingly, fear. Fear made it impossible for me to read the document and understand how my insured car being in a crash eight weeks ago had led to this arriving on my doorstep. My brain spiraled out of control. I saw words like "prison," and before I could stop myself, I was envisioning my whole world falling apart. Shaking, heart racing, feeling sick and fuzzy in my head and my mouth, I phoned my insurance company. I'll never forget the kindness of the woman who answered the phone. She heard and understood I was extremely distressed, even if my story was a bit jumbled. She seemed genuinely concerned and caring. She told me to take a few deep breaths and to put the kettle on while she looked into it for me. Immediately, I felt myself settle. I did what she said, then returned to the call. She talked me reassuringly through the next steps (I had phoned the wrong insurance company in my panic!), acknowledged the stress I was feeling and did not dismiss it. She didn't catastrophize, or tell me it was going to be OK; she didn't shame me or make me feel judged. She was just a warm person who connected to me as a human being and wasn't afraid to offer me support, even if she couldn't fix the problem.

The gratitude I felt was overwhelming. Thanks to her, I was quickly calm enough to sort out the problem. Twenty-four hours later, I learned that the court papers were a process to get my insurance company to settle for a higher amount. It turned out to be a storm in a teacup.

Two things I took away from this experience:

1. Sometimes the things that create the biggest fear response in us are not physical threat experiences (e.g., the car crash). Instead, they are words, imagined possibilities, not understanding whether something does or does not jeopardize our safety and security. In my memory, the car crash was less stressful than the few hours of fear I experienced after receiving the court papers.

2. A complete stranger connected with me authentically in the moment I was most vulnerable and, in doing this, had the power to soothe my fear within a minute and help me get back on track to resolve my difficulties.

We will explore point one further in chapter 8. In this chapter, we will be looking into point two: the power of connection before correction (a term developed by many esteemed professionals in this area including Dan Siegel, Tina Payne Bryson, Kim Golding, Dan Hughes, and Bruce Perry).[26]

> ☁ **Reflection Box**
>
> Think of a time you and another person have both been in emotional distress. How did it feel? What was the outcome of the conversation? Or think of a time when you've flipped your lid about a problem and the other person has rushed in with all the solutions.
>
> Now think of a time when you've flipped your lid, but the other person has really connected with you, and given you those few seconds of feeling understood. How did it feel different? Were you then able to move on collaboratively to think about any possible resolutions?

The window of tolerance

In order to understand the power of connection, we need to go back to a bit more brain science. Dan Siegel developed the concept of the "window of tolerance."[27] This is the sweet spot where we're stimulated enough that our upstairs (thinking) brain and downstairs (emotional) brain are nicely connected. We're not overstimulated or stressed to the point that we become so distressed that we can't think clearly or engage in new learning.

Take a look at the illustration of the window of tolerance. When we're in the white part of the window of tolerance, we're emotionally regulated. We're able to connect with others, feel a range of feelings and make good decisions, as our downstairs (emotional) and upstairs (thinking) brains are connected and working well together. As described in the previous chapter, this is the place we want to support our children to get to when they are experiencing distress.

When we become dysregulated, the diagram illustrates how we can go in two directions. In the dark gray window you can see we can become **hyper**aroused (like I did as soon as I opened the brown envelope). This activates our autonomic nervous system to enable our bodies to respond well to danger (see chapter 7 where this is covered in detail in relation to anxiety). In these (flip-the-lid) moments, our bodies and minds are racing to take flight or confront the problem. Our feelings are exaggerated.

HYPERAROUSAL (TOO MUCH ENERGY)

Fight or flight: shouting, running away, hyperalert, racing body and mind, not listening to others

Feels like: rage, panic, fear, excitement

No new learning can happen

OPTIMAL LEVEL OF AROUSAL – WINDOW OF TOLERANCE (OPTIMAL ENERGY)

Self-control: aware of self, others, space, time

Can feel: the full range of feelings

New learning can happen

HYPOAROUSAL (TOO LITTLE ENERGY)

Freeze: exhausted, tired, slow, drained, shut down

Feels like: flat, no emotions/feelings, numb, dissociated

No new learning can happen

The Window of Tolerance

Alternatively, we can go in the other direction and become **hypo**aroused (pale gray window). This is where the autonomic nervous system shuts down (discussed in more detail in chapter 10 in relation to low mood). Everything slows down and becomes an effort. Rather than feeling too much, we may feel nothing at all.

In chapter 4, we explored the situations when you or your child might be triggered (flipped lid) into the dark gray or pale gray window. In this chapter, I share the tools you need to help your child get from the dark or pale gray window to the white window (from flipped lid to a connected upstairs and downstairs brain).

It's good to talk: Right time, right place (for you and for them)

I'm picking my daughter up from school after a long day at work and the second she gets in the car, she launches into a tirade of anger and frustration at her day, telling me: "So and so did this . . . now my name is in the book . . . I'm going to get a detention and it's not fair." I'm fuming. Why do drama and my daughter always seem to go together? In her rants, everyone else is the problem and she doesn't take any responsibility for her own behavior. I try to offer the teacher's point of view, explaining rules are rules. This seems to agitate her more and, before we know it, we're both hyperaroused (flipping our lids). By the time we get home, she's storming off to her bedroom, "hating" me as well. I feel like I'm a terrible mom, exasperated and wishing for an escape from parenthood altogether, knowing it's going to be a long evening.

As this scenario demonstrates, the biggest mistake I make as a parent is seeing my kids worked up about something and moving immediately to problem-solving, or trying to resolve the situation. I'm so focused on getting through the tasks of the day that sorting things as quickly and painlessly as possible is often my main priority. However, typically when I do this, my children respond with further difficult behaviors or increased distress. I've learned that just taking a few seconds to pause and shift my attention onto what I'm seeing in my child is a powerful tool, and one that can make them feel like I want to connect with their world, and in so doing, "engage, don't enrage," to quote Siegel and Payne Bryson.[28]

No matter their age, our children value more than anything our undivided attention and feeling properly listened to. When they feel distressed or confused, having someone listen to them and validate their difficult feelings without judgment helps them feel comforted and safe. We know this as parents, but ironically, we also know that when our stress levels go up, our emotional availability typically goes down, making it harder to be responsive to our children's needs in those moments they often need us most. If we want to tune in to our children, it's essential we're aware of our own window of tolerance, as we likely need to be in the sweet (white) spot to get the best outcomes for us and our children when strong feelings are involved.

Connection before correction: Notice, connect, validate, collaborate

Many experts in the area of child development have described the principles and process of connecting with a child before moving to solutions/correction.[29] These experts have outlined the key components necessary to support our children back into their window of tolerance, or unflipping their lid. This method helps us as parents balance the tricky challenge of providing empathy and warmth, as well as boundaries and structure.

These four simple steps—notice, connect, validate, then correct (I prefer the word "collaborate")—can transform a high-stress moment into an opportunity to develop problem-solving skills, as well as learning about appropriate rules and boundaries and agreeing consequences.

We don't have to do this all the time; we just have to repeat it enough that our children can start developing the skills. Although at first following these steps might feel unnatural and more effortful than your usual response, in time it will get easier, feel more normal, and save time, helping to de-escalate situations that might usually lead to more time-consuming difficulties.

1. Notice

What is happening for your child right now, from their perspective? What is happening for you right now? How are you feeling? Is your lid about to flip? What can you do to regulate yourself? If you notice yourself feeling overwhelmed, try: (1) breathing deeply (breathing exercises on page 155), (2) stepping away, and/or (3) asking for help from someone you trust (your partner, older sibling).

2. Connect

Stay calm. Keep your body language and facial expressions relaxed and use your voice to show interest or care. Remember, you're trying to soothe the downstairs brain. Come down to your child's level (e.g., if they are little, crouch on the floor. If they are sitting down, sit down alongside them) and be physically present without imposing yourself on them. Give them a bit of space to transition into a conversation. Sometimes our children benefit from physical touch, a hug or patting their back. Sometimes our children won't want this. Use your knowledge about your child to guide you. Children may need space or a reduction in sensory information to help them regulate, such as being in a quieter environment or having access to a weighted blanket/sensory sleeping bag.

3. Validate

We don't have an emotional X-ray, so we can't know what feelings are going on in others' heads. What we can do is imagine and use this curiosity to listen attentively, without judgment, to encourage our children to share more about what's going on in their world. Be careful not to impose your view on your child. Listen to their reality in the moment without trying to solve the problem or denying their feelings (or defending yourself!). Allowing our children to be truly heard is one of the most powerful experiences we can give them, and by doing this, we can **"name it to tame it,"** in the words of Dr. Siegel. By compassionately recognizing some of the things our children might be feeling, we can help them feel understood, and guide them in learning how to make links between words and feelings (connecting the downstairs and upstairs brain), building their emotional literacy. Some examples of this include: "I'm wondering if you're feeling sad because you've missed your friends this weekend?"; "This homework seems really hard; I can see why you might be fed up and cross." Or: "I wonder if your brother pushing you has made you feel angry? It doesn't feel fair."

These words are supporting the downstairs/upstairs brain connection. Speaking out loud, compassionately and curiously, what might be going on for our child helps them feel understood and if we're curious rather than sure, they may correct us and give us more information to help make sense of what's going on for them.

4. Collaborate

Once our children's lids are back on and they feel heard and validated, you're both likely to be in a good space to use the upstairs brain to collaborate to resolve the challenge. For example: "Is there a chance next week for you to have a friend over?"; "Do you want a break from your homework, then we could maybe look at it together?"; "I'm going to talk to your brother about what happened; he shouldn't have pushed you. What could you do next time you and him are about to get into a fight?"

When you're in the collaborative zone with your child, come up with ideas together to help for the next time they feel overwhelmed. For example: "Do you think being somewhere quieter helps? Would it have helped if I had given you a few minutes on your own?" This final stage of collaboration is where your child's connection between the downstairs and upstairs brain is growing, supporting them to learn essential life skills to both feel and resolve problems. It's also a place where you and your child build trust and respect in your relationship and recognize the value of thinking together.

It might feel like you need a lot of time to do this four-step process. But depending on the situation it usually doesn't. For example, with the earlier-described collecting-my-daughter-from-school scenario, the four steps could have looked like this:

Step 1: Notice

Pay attention to my own stress response to my daughter's story—*this is pressing my buttons, beware of how I'm going to react.* Notice this is a difficult time of day for both of us (tired and hungry). Notice she's really upset and unlikely to listen to anything I have to say right now.

Step 2: Connect

Focus on driving, but have relaxed, interested body language (non-verbal cues like nodding my head and having a concerned face), so she can see I'm listening.

Step 3: Validate

Say something that shows I have put myself in her shoes, like: "Wow, it sounds like a difficult day, and I guess you're worried about missing lunch break tomorrow if you have a detention."

Step 4: Collaborate

Prompt this by asking, "Shall we talk more about this after dinner? I reckon we're both pretty tired and hungry right now. It's been a long day for both of us."

ACTIVITY BOX

As we manage the tricky balance between being caring and disciplining our children, we may find ourselves in the habit of reacting in some of the ways below. Tick the "correction-before-connection" traps that you feel you rely on more heavily:

- ✔ ignoring or invalidating (e.g., "It's not a big deal, you shouldn't be this upset");

- ✔ giving negative attention (e.g., shouting);

- ✔ threatening a punishment as a consequence of the current behavior (e.g., "You'll have your phone taken away");

- ✔ providing an immediate solution to the problem (e.g., "Just tell your friend you're not going");

- ✔ doing a task for your child or giving into their demand (e.g., child has an outburst when asked to unload the dishwasher, so you do it yourself and don't ask the next time);

- ✔ distracting (e.g., giving a treat to occupy them or letting them watch something);
- ✔ imposing more rules (e.g., "Right, you're going to bed early");
- ✔ declaring consequences that are disproportionate and unexpected (e.g., "I'm getting rid of your phone/games console").

These will be things we do while juggling life's pressures and our own internal world. As a parent, I often find that I'm responding to my children's flipped lids in the above ways in situations when they are being non-compliant, I need them to be cooperative, and I'm short of time and patience (e.g., on a busy school run, in a public place, resisting going to bed). In these tricky moments as parents we often need a quick fix. However, what feels like a quick fix can often lead to further challenges, which in the long run end up taking more time and energy (e.g., our child's distress further escalates into more difficult behaviors).

Although these correction-before-connection traps are a natural part of parenting, if we get stuck in over-relying on them, we miss opportunities to help support our children to learn healthier ways to understand and deal with feelings (strengthen the connection between the upstairs and downstairs brain). Let's revisit the Johnsons to see how they might use the four-step model to break free from the correction-before-connection trap.

- -

CASE STUDY

Bella's Story (Part 2)

Back to the Johnsons. Once I explained the window of tolerance to them and the four steps—notice, connect, validate and collaborate—to help Bella reconnect her downstairs and upstairs brain they were able to try this approach on a Sunday night when Bella came home from her dad's. This is what it looked like.

Notice
Mom noticed that when Bella came home from her dad's, she was uneasy and uncommunicative. She tuned into how this made her feel: worried that Bella didn't want to be at home with her, worried that Bella might explode and the family night would be ruined. Mom took a few deep breaths to calm down her downstairs brain.

Connect
Mom came and sat with Bella while she played her computer game. She showed a positive interest in her game. She kept her body language relaxed and her voice quiet and calm. Bella said she wasn't feeling great.

Validate
Mom put herself in Bella's shoes and was curious. She said, "I'm guessing it must be hard coming home from Dad's; I wonder if you feel sad leaving Dad?" Bella replied, "Kind of. Except it's like this guilt feeling I get—that I'm happy to be home, but I know my dad would be upset if he knew that. But it gets stuck in my throat—all these feelings."

Mom gave a bit of space, then replied, "That sounds really tough. It makes sense this would feel hard. I'm sorry I haven't always helped with this when you get home. Me getting cross probably makes you feel worse." Mom paused. "I wonder if there is anything your stepdad and I can do to help it feel a bit easier when you get home and your downstairs brain is mixed up with difficult feelings?" Bella was quick to reply, "I just need a bit of time to zone out, I think. I feel everyone wants me to be happy that I'm home and just fit back in, and I find that pressure difficult."

Collaborate
At this point Bella (and her mom) are thinking and feeling, meaning they can think together about how to help with the transition from Dad's house to Mom's house. In this space, Bella asked that when she got home she had at least forty-five minutes of time doing an activity of her choice without interruption, just to help her relax into being back at home and settle into the new routine with a sense of autonomy. Bella and her mom worked out

that coming to the family meal was really tricky for Bella on Sunday nights, so they made a plan that her and Mom would spend some time together after the others had finished eating, making a sandwich and watching a TV show Bella liked together. This helped Bella feel part of the family, without feeling she was letting them down. Bella and Mom agreed to the plan and tried it the following time Bella came home from her dad's. They found that things were much easier for everyone. We'll look at what happens next in chapter 6.

The power of Sorry

As parents we can get it wrong. Sometimes, our downstairs brain might take over and lead us to overreact, or say things we don't mean. It's OK to make mistakes as parents—it helps prepare our children for relationships in the real world, where others are likely to make mistakes too. The most important thing is to be aware when we **do** get it wrong and ensure that when we get the opportunity, we reach out to our child to acknowledge how we might have got it wrong, and repair our relationship with them. Finding the right time to say sorry is vital. The collaborative zone is a good time to apologize and make any repairs in the relationship, just like Bella's mom managed to in her story.

Many of the young people I work with value genuine parental apologies. They learn that getting it wrong, and acknowledging this, is a helpful way to stay connected with others and build strong relationships. Your child is much more likely to learn the value of saying sorry if they've experienced how to do it well from you. Take a look at the activity box below for how to prepare for successful noticing, connecting, validating, and collaborating.

ACTIVITY BOX

Right Time, Right Place, Right Pace

Practice in low-stake situations

Plan a time when you know you can try this four-stage approach. When learning new skills, it's best to develop them in low-stress contexts. Prepare for success by planning a time of the day and situation when you're likely to be feeling most resourced to notice more of what's going on for your child.

Creating a pause with curiosity

Building in a pause to slow everything down can make a huge difference when things are getting heated—even three deep breaths can be enough. Putting a space between the itch (your child shouting at you) and the scratch (you feeling angry and shouting back) can create room to notice more of what might be happening. Controlling your attention by pausing can lead to a different response from you— one that will support your child (and you) in connecting the upstairs and downstairs brain.

Planned connection time

Sometimes, we recognize we need to create a safe space to talk with our children about difficult things. When we think something is wrong, or are dealing with an earlier problem (e.g., difficult behavior or a family event), we might directly approach our children, asking "What's wrong?" or "We need to talk about the consequences for your bad behavior earlier," which often doesn't get the response we're looking for. In my experience, we're much more likely to build connection and opportunity to talk about more difficult stuff if we engage with our child at a time when they're doing an activity where they are relaxed, e.g., sitting alongside them when they're watching their TV show and taking a genuine, non-judgmental, quiet interest. In these less-confrontational moments, our child/adolescent is more likely to open up about what's going on for them. Whether it's on a car journey together, going for a walk, cooking, or playing with them, it's about taking a chance to join their world and sit alongside them, giving them some control. If there's a need to discuss consequences for difficult behavior, asking your child when might be a good time to talk it through helpfully (both in the white zone) will set your conversation up for success (e.g., "Shall we talk about what happened this morning after dinner, when things are a bit quieter? We can have a chat over a walk with the dog or while I'm tidying up the kitchen if that feels like a good time for you?"). These are the interpersonal skills we would like to see in our children as they grow into adulthood and learn to negotiate relationships in their world.

Preparing for success:
Understanding vulnerabilities

It's important that we have appropriate expectations for our children, especially if they've experienced difficulties in the past or have developmental or neurodevelopmental diversity. Often when I meet with families, I discover that a parent wrongly assumes that their child (a) has understood what's expected of them or the task, and (b) has the skills to complete the task. Often difficult behaviors emerge when either or both of these assumptions are incorrect.

As parents, understanding our children's vulnerabilities helps us provide an environment where we can support skills development, rather than making them feel like they are never getting it right, or permanently in trouble. Children can get stuck in a cycle of feeling down about themselves, and may build up lots of defenses to protect against further failure (e.g., not attempting to do new things). Some young people struggle more with emotional regulation tasks and consequently need more support from the adults around them. The possible reasons for this in relation to trauma are explained in the Fact Box on the next page.

Structure, routine and consistency are particularly helpful for all young people, but likely even more so for those with neurodevelopmental differences or who have experienced a history of trauma. Finding ways to increase the level of continuity, structure, and routine your child has in their life can help support emotional regulation.

Trauma: What happened to us?

Some people's downstairs brains are especially sensitive and can be triggered more easily (meaning they have a narrower window of tolerance). This may be caused by something traumatic that happened in their life, or needed experiences they did not have. For example, if we go back to Bella's story, when she was a young child, her parents' struggles and events in their own lives made it difficult for them to care for Bella. She also witnessed domestic violence. Bella did not have an available parent to help her make sense of her feelings. Instead, she learned to hide her feelings so as not to increase her parents' distress or risk them withdrawing from her. Bella's experiences as a child meant, in order to survive, her brain became more sensitive to looking out for danger.

Children who have experienced traumatic events in their lives are more likely to need support from others, whether these traumas are associated with key relationships during periods of development (like Bella), or one-off traumatic events.

For these children, their downstairs/upstairs brain age may not mirror their chronological age. Bella may need support from others to regulate her emotions more like a five-year-old would, rather than a twelve-year-old, helping her develop these skills to move her closer to her age.

I help parents and school staff to think about some of the things they might do to support a child if they were five, not twelve, and ask them to try some of these things out. This support for these young people is like filling in the gaps to give them the tools they need so they can catch up with their peer group. You can't expect a child to read if they've not learned the alphabet; you would teach them the alphabet. Sadly, particularly in high school education settings, when children present with difficult behaviors that may be representative of an emotional regulation skills deficit, they are punished (through exclusion or detention), rather than given the opportunity to learn or feel loved and valued, thus perpetuating the cycle of adverse experiences.

It's important not to shame children who may need more support in this area. Shame brings out our children's self-protection—which could be withdrawal or attacking others (see the shield of shame in chapter 6), which can make it harder to build connection and opportunities to support them in developing these skills.

The brain's ability to be flexible and adaptable and grow through learning is an incredible thing. It means that if we practice the skills of noticing, connecting, validating and collaborating with our children, their window of tolerance will expand and their brains will improve their ability to integrate emotions and thinking. The more opportunities we have to do this, the stronger the connections and our children's brains will become. Just like how often we go to the gym, experiencing things regularly and consistently is key to helping our children regulate their emotions, and every interaction we and others have with them is an opportunity to practice this. Try to fit it in once or twice a week if you can, and remember: little and often.

ACTIVITY BOX

We all have five senses, which are critical in communicating with both our downstairs and upstairs brain: sight, smell, touch, hearing, and taste. Another route to both dysregulation and regulation is through sensory information (think about how powerful a piece of music, or a particular smell might be for your mood or memories). Some children may have sensory sensitivities that impact their emotional regulation. Others may have earlier trauma that is triggered by sensory information. Finding ways of using the range of senses to support regulation can be helpful, and means we don't need to rely solely on language to communicate.

You can do this by helping your child make a **sensory box**. You can even make one for yourself. Get an empty shoebox and with your child find items they experience as calming in moments of feeling overwhelmed or dysregulated. These could include different textured fabrics or objects (even fidget toys); music or items that make different sounds; smell-evoking objects like perfume; visual items like photos of important people, pets, or places; or items that can be tasted. This box is something children can decorate and keep in a safe place and go to independently to help regulate themselves.

SUMMARY

→ The window of tolerance is the sweet spot where we can communicate well with others, listen and learn, as well as feel a healthy range of emotions (our upstairs and downstairs brain are connected). There are times when we step out of the window of tolerance and become hyperaroused or hypoaroused (flip the lid).

Both of these states feel unpleasant and make it difficult to communicate and learn.

→ Helping our children (or ourselves) move from being hyperaroused or hypoaroused into the window of tolerance is most effective if we can find ways to connect with them.

→ Connecting with our children involves keeping an awareness of our own emotional responses, finding ways to not be overwhelmed ourselves, and then following these four steps: notice, connect, validate, collaborate.

→ Some children and adults may have a smaller window of tolerance, due to their biology (genetics), neurodevelopmental diversity, or traumatic events they've experienced. It's important that we use these tools to support these young people (and adults) with the opportunity to build skills to help grow their window of tolerance.

→ We're sensory creatures. It's helpful for our brains to attach words to emotions. It's also helpful to use our senses to support ourselves toward the window of tolerance when we might be distressed.

Chapter 6
Working out what's important

One of the biggest challenges for me as a parent is seeing my children in pain, whether that is physical or emotional. Some elements of physical pain can sometimes feel more managable because, after years of being a parent, I more or less know what I need to do (e.g., cold compress, paracetamol, plaster, sick bowl, cuddles, staying calm and attentive). If I'm really confused or worried, I can call a medical help line for advice, make an appointment with my family doctor or, in an emergency, call an ambulance or go to an emergency department.

Emotional pain is a whole different world. As with physical pain, we want to protect our children from emotional discomfort. We may protect our children from this because we don't want them to go through what we may have as a young person. It's likely that we find our own emotional discomfort or pain something we try to avoid. When my children's dad and I broke up, it was almost unbearable to see my children suffering emotionally as I went through my own rollercoaster of feelings.

It's natural that when we see our children in pain, we want to take it away or reduce it. Unfortunately, it's one of life's paradoxes that in order to experience life fully, we need to experience the full spectrum of emotions. We may not want our children to endure feelings of sadness, anger, envy, or shame, and yet a part of us knows that in order to navigate life and truly value the feelings of joy and happiness, they will have to. If we don't feel sadness, how do we know what it means to lose something precious? Without anger, who would stand up to injustice? Unlike a broken leg or split lip, emotions that create discomfort are a necessary and inevitable part of being human, and an important part of developing who we are, what we value and our moral compass.

The good, the bad, and the not-so-ugly . . .

It's easy to fall into the trap of seeing certain emotions as "good" or "bad." This is particularly true for our adolescents, who are growing up surrounded by social media messaging that promotes "happiness" as if it's something everyone experiences continuously. Having difficult feelings is often portrayed as having failed and, as parents, we may unintentionally reinforce this, especially if seeing our children in this state creates strong emotions in us.

We all know that Facebook and Instagram posts are full of our own friends' stories and photos showing off the best bits of their lives. Even if we're aware of the reality (e.g., the person posting was arguing with their other half just before they uploaded a happy photo of them both), it's still hard not to get sucked into the façade, comparing our lives to others' portrayals of theirs. Even posts where people describe the level of adversity they are miraculously managing so positively can unintentionally make us feel even more inadequate or guilty about the concerns we have.

It would be wonderful to work toward a culture where we could see emotions as a helpful signpost to what matters to us and support for understanding ourselves better, enabling us to use these emotions wisely. In this chapter, we'll explore how we do this with our children.

The emotional x-ray

When our child is in physical pain, we observe their physical symptoms (e.g., temperature, visible damage, acuity of pain) and ask questions—"Where's the pain? What kind of pain? Do you feel sick?" These observations are our attempt to work out the underlying cause of our child's physical symptoms and, most importantly, to establish what the best treatment for help is, if required. It might be that the illness will pass with the body's immune system simply needing time to do its job. It could just benefit from rest and perhaps a painkiller (e.g., a cold virus, chicken pox, a blister). Other times, there may be something that requires treatment in order for the body to heal properly or stop a deterioration in health (e.g., appendicitis, badly broken limb, bacterial infection). As a parent, your anxiety about your child's physical symptoms is to ensure that you take the necessary action for your child to receive the appropriate treatment. You wouldn't want to use a painkiller to mask something that needed treatment and, left untreated, could be life-threatening (e.g., meningitis), or impact your child's recovery from an injury (e.g., a broken limb that requires a cast/surgery).

Unfortunately, we don't have an emotional X-ray and therefore, it's harder to take this same approach with emotional discomfort or pain. We may see the symptoms of distress (e.g., crying, moodiness, withdrawal, not eating, self-harm). We might feel confused or have our own emotional response (just like when we see physical discomfort or pain) of anxiety or worry. We could ask what's wrong or guess something is wrong, but we don't necessarily have the tools or vocabulary to discover what the underlying cause of the pain could be, what it means, and the best course of action. Perhaps we unintentionally suggest the equivalent of a painkiller (e.g., distraction, watch a screen, have a treat, focus on the positives, "it will be alright") to mask a problem that our child needs more help to understand, rather than distract away from or ignore. By doing this, we may accidentally reinforce the idea that emotional discomfort is something to be avoided if possible.

Research has shown that those who are able to notice and tolerate their emotions do better in terms of their wellbeing.[30] If we're able to learn to tune into strong emotions, we can discover they may be telling us something about (a) what's important to us and (b) what's happening in our life. By understanding this, we can try to establish what needs to change and if we need help from others to support that change.

As parents, we can play a crucial role in supporting our children with:

* becoming more emotionally aware;
* helping them turn toward, rather than run away from or block, painful emotions;
* learning how to understand how emotions might give information about what's most important to us.

We can do this through sitting with the feelings alongside our children, exploring values, and using them to guide us on what to do next. I'll explain each of these in more detail here.

Sitting with the feelings

When my then nine-year-old daughter heard the news that her dad was having a baby with his new partner, she was initially really excited. Having two brothers, she began to consider life with a baby sister and not being the only girl in the family. Around a week after she received the news, I found her crying in her bed after I thought she had gone to sleep. I crept into her bed in the dark and lay with her. "What's up?" I asked. She said it was about the new baby between sobs. She didn't want Dad to have a new baby. She might not like it. With my emotional guess-ray, I wondered if she might feel sad, angry, insecure (fearful of rejection) and possibly a little envy, as this baby would be with Dad every day of the week.

With a bit more reassurance that I was hearing her and not judging her, she went on to explain she was scared that having a new baby would mean her dad would love her less, that she would stop being so special to him. In fact, she asked, was it possible he could stop loving her at all, especially as the new baby would be with him all the time? For me, these had been all of my fears when I heard the news, so it took a lot of internal resource to put aside how I was feeling, and instead focus on what my daughter needed right now. I couldn't take away this pain, I couldn't guarantee she wouldn't struggle with some of the things she was starting to worry about. I wanted to be able to offer all the solutions, tell her it would be fine, to not be silly. I'd talk to her dad and make sure this wouldn't happen. But I didn't. I lay there, bearing the pain (which was crushing me, too), but staying calm and loving, sitting with it so she didn't need to feel afraid or ashamed of it. Honoring her world, her experience. For a long time, I lay with her in the dark, our arms touching, hearing her cry and feeling her rapid breathing; my quiet presence eventually soothed her.

Many years after this experience, I listened to a podcast with professor and author Brené Brown, where she talked about a similar incident with her teenage daughter experiencing a break-up with her boyfriend. She, like me, had sat on her daughter's bed, in the dark, wanting to take away the pain her daughter was going through. The whole time she was looking at the light switch on the wall thinking, "This is so hard; I just want to turn on that light and take away the pain." But she didn't. She understood sitting with her daughter in the dark at that moment was her main task as parent.

So often we do not want our children to experience difficult emotions. Instead, we want to take them away or solve the problem. But learning to go through this emotion and understanding it's safe to do this can help a young person develop resilience and a sense that when hard things happen, they have the skills to deal with it. As parents, we don't have to pretend we know everything or that we're always in control. The key is to show up, see our children, and provide them with the reassurance that we can find a way through this challenge, even if it does hurt.

As described in chapter 5, when our children are in distress, the first thing we need to do is sit alongside them and acknowledge their feelings without trying to move them too quickly from the pain they're in. When experiencing distress, it's a vulnerable moment, and many of us may feel especially sensitive to the rejection of others. If, in our vulnerable moments, we feel misunderstood or sense we're likely to be hurt further, we may throw up the shield of shame (see the illustration below), leading to behaviors that push others away, right at the point we most need connection and care. If a child feels seen and understood, this will immediately lead to the lowering of the shield of shame (soothing the downstairs brain and connecting the upstairs brain). A child will then be in a better place to take on thinking, talking, and/or making sense of what now, what next.

That night in my daughter's bed, it was hard for me because I was also in emotional pain. But I was able to comfort my daughter by sitting with her feelings and showing my care for her in my body language and presence. I was honest about the fact that I couldn't solve the problem or take away the pain; that I didn't have all the answers for some really tough stuff. In doing this, I supported my daughter to feel that despite so much uncertainty, her feelings were understandable and bearable. I was able to help her understand that (a) her feelings are important and (b) that she can cope with the uncertainty of her changing world.

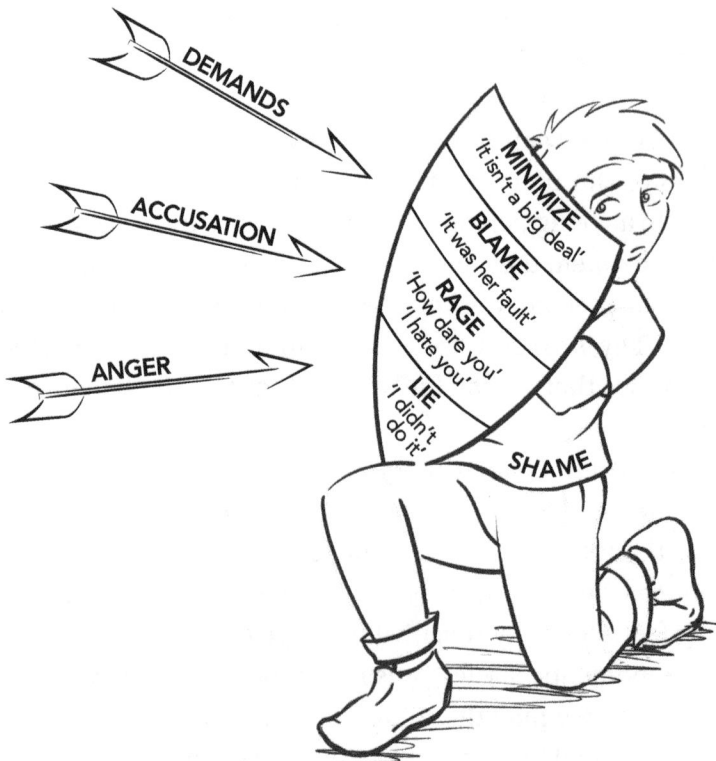

The Shield of Shame (adapted from Golding and Hughes, 2012)[31]

Fact Box

A disproportionate response can be a clue to unresolved trauma. Strong emotions that can overwhelm or pop up at unexpected times could be linked to difficult memories or events in your or your child's past that have had a big impact on you/ them.[32] You/they may not have fully made sense of or healed from those events, and you might be surprised by disproportionate responses to certain types of events. You may feel confused as to why, for example, witnessing a family member argue or a friend not returning a message can trigger a flood of irrational fear or even lead to a feeling of dissociation. Trying to make the links and increase your awareness of how your past losses or challenges may influence your current emotional responses can help signpost to whether you/your child might need more time for healing and perhaps getting the support from another trusted person (or professional) to talk through these unresolved memories or traumas.

Edith Eger, a Holocaust survivor, has written one of the most inspiring books I've ever read: The Gift. *There's a line in it that has stayed with me: "When we don't allow ourselves to grieve our losses, wounds, and disappointments, we're doomed to keep reliving them."[33] Increasing your awareness when painful emotions come up for you or your children can help with creating space to talk about difficult events and lead to healing.*

Exploring the underlying values

Our emotions show us what's important and signpost us to our values. So when we or our children experience a strong emotion it can be helpful to ask, *What value is that emotion signposting us to?* For example, if your child is feeling angry and sad about an event that has felt rejecting (perhaps they weren't invited to a friend's party), this could signpost to your child's desire for belonging and friendship. Essentially, these difficult moments give an opportunity to help your child identify who they are and why they care.

ACTIVITY BOX

Look at the list of values below (you can refer to a more extensive list on Brené Brown's website).[34] Choose three from the list that you feel are most important to you, and that you aim to live your life by. Alternatively, come up with your own if you can think of ones more suitable than those listed.

Choose three values that you think might be important to your child. Are you surprised by how similar or different they might be? What does this tell you about what are likely to be: (1) your priorities in life and (2) your child's?

To complete this activity with your child, write out these values on pieces of paper to make a pile of cards. Ask your young person to look through the cards with you and pick out the cards that reflect the three values that are most important to them right now. They might want to create their own cards. Explore together what's important to them about the values they've picked.

Loving	Being loved	Achievement	Connection	Belonging
Security	Friendship	Creativity	Passion	Movement
Adventure	Learning	Curiosity	Knowledge	Nature
Respect	Discipline	Pride	Freedom	Forgiveness
Fun	Community	Humor	Home	Fairness
Safety	Trust	Growth	Diversity	Family

Helping my daughter work out the values underlying her feelings

Going back to that night described above, after sitting with my daughter's pain, we were then able to think together about what her feelings might be telling her, which bits to listen to, and which bits to challenge (our thoughts are not always facts: see chapter 8 for more on this). Her upstairs brain and downstairs brain were working well together with my help.

I said to her, "This is tricky. I'm sorry I can't make it better or tell you what will happen but I think what you're saying is that being loved by your dad is one of the most important things of all right now. So, I'm guessing this new baby makes you feel scared that Dad's love might run out or go in just the direction of the new baby, which makes sense that would make you feel sad and scared because you love your dad so much."

"Yes," she nodded.

"I wonder if this fear is true, or just telling you how important your dad's love is to you?" I went on. "Remember when your third baby cousin was born? It was so exciting; he was so cute—you're so good at helping look after him. Do you love him?"

"Yes, I do, very much," she said.

"What about his two older brothers, do you love them less since he was born?" I continued.

"No!" she said. "That would be impossible and totally unfair."

"So," I asked, curiously. "Do you think that means when new important people come along you can make more love in your heart, or do you think you only have so much love to give in your life?"

"No, I can grow more love," she answered.

I continued, "Do you think you'll grow more love for your baby brother or sister?"

"Yes, of course," she responded.

"Do you think your dad will grow more love too, or take it away from you? Remember, he loved your older brother before you were born?"

"He can grow more love," she said with a newfound certainty.

We then went on to explore how she could let her dad know this was a worry, so he could make sure that he did not unintentionally reinforce this fear in some of the ways he might respond to his changing family. Earlier on, she had talked about not seeing him that weekend. Following our discussion, we were able to work out that this course of action was based on fear, rather than helping her feel loved by her dad, which is what she wanted. She recognized she might need more quality time with him for a while, not less.

Moving toward what's important: The moral compass

By exploring the values behind emotions, not only do we discover what's happening in our lives that might be undermining what's important to us, we can also use this approach to help create a space between an event that might have triggered a strong feeling—and what we do next. This enables us to not only feel a sense of control and choice over our behaviors, but also helps to consider what we can do next to move toward what's important to us rather than away from it. This may not only help us resolve some of the challenges in our life which are creating the difficult emotions, but also ensures we're intentionally supporting ourselves move in the direction of our moral compass. This ultimately improves our emotional agility and our sense of wellbeing, making us better people to be around. We can support our children to do the same thing in our connected, collaborative conversations with them.

For example, if your child is angry because they lost in a football game, they might benefit from being supported (coached) to consider what value the emotion is pointing to (e.g., being the best, sportsmanship, teamwork). You can then explore what they might do next to honor the value (e.g., focus on what to work on for next time, behave in a sportsman-like way, lean into their team, praise them for effort), rather than what their anger might urge them to do (e.g., give up playing, not shake the opposition's hand or minimize their win, withdraw or blame their teammates). This process encourages tolerating difficult feelings and also considering ways to encourage the growth of our children into well-rounded young people who, with the help of both their upstairs and downstairs brains, can make wise choices about how they live their lives and respond in difficult situations. Take a look at the table on page 131 for some examples that can guide conversations you could have with your child.

CASE STUDY

Bella's Story (Part 3)

What's most important to Bella?

With Bella's parents, we used the values cards (see page 124) to help Bella discover her most important values right now. These were: **loving and being loved, belonging, loyalty, and feeling safe and secure.** Based on these values, Bella and her mom could see how Sunday nights were often so triggering for her, especially when others were cross with her. When she felt explosive rage on Sunday nights, she recognized it was because she was afraid that her mom and stepdad felt she was a let-down and that they wouldn't want her to live with them anymore. She wanted to feel part of the family when she got home, but she found herself feeling too many tricky feelings to be able to settle with everyone. Understanding what was important to Bella enabled the family to come up with a plan that would support her downstairs and upstairs brain to stay connected, and would also help her do things that moved her toward her values (e.g., having some guilt-free space when she first got home, and then having time with Mom eating some dinner and watching a TV show), instead of away from her values (e.g., shouting and hitting out at others, isolating herself).

Because the family had talked about and sat with their feelings, they understood that Bella wasn't deliberately trying to be difficult, or wishing she hadn't come home. Rather, she was processing some difficult feelings. Bella also understood her parents' values (loving and being loved, respect, discipline and family) and that when they got upset with her behavior it wasn't that they did not love her; instead they were worried about what it meant for them as a family and her happiness, now and in the future. Her parents considered the things they could do to move toward their values (e.g., providing space for understanding, communicating kindly) rather than away (e.g., being quick to anger, shouting, giving unexpected sanctions).

Going forward, Sunday nights became more relaxed for everyone and the difficult behaviors disappeared. Bella and her parents' relationship grew and she was able to share more about her feelings, as well as giving them a heads up if her downstairs brain was about to flip the lid. Bella's parents understood she might need help to work out her feelings and talk about them. They created more protected time for these opportunities and did more curious talking out loud about what might be going on. By respecting Bella's space, Bella learned to self-regulate and become less dependent on the rules of the house being the main guide for her behavior (she started listening to her moral compass).

Bella felt happier because the important things to her—loving and being loved, belonging, loyalty, feeling safe and secure—were being honored in the family time they spent together and she no longer feared her distressed behavior would lead to losing her family. Her parents felt happier because as a family they spent more time honoring the things that were important to them: loving and being loved, respect, discipline, and family. By understanding the Brain House, learning to connect, validating each other's experiences, and doing more of the things that mattered, their family was a happier and more fulfilling place to be, despite the difficult feelings.

- -

Noticing what's important

One of the things that helped Bella's family shift the focus away from the problem toward understanding what's important was them getting better at noticing Bella behaving in ways that were consistent with her own and/or the family values.

A simple way of doing this on a daily basis is noticing what our children seem to value and describing this out loud, for example, "I notice you working really hard to help your friends; you must really care about friendship and belonging" or "Thank you for being so helpful and kind to your brother by bringing him his bag; it shows me you care about family." Even the tiniest hints of something we might consider a value, we can describe out loud to reinforce what we hope to see more of in our families, rather than noticing what we *don't* see (e.g., "You never help me out round the house") or focusing on what we see that we don't like ("You're always saying mean things to your brother"). By paying attention positively we do two things: (1) encourage more of these behaviors and (2) build our child's sense of self-esteem.

Wisdom

When we bring together the downstairs (emotional brain) and the upstairs (thinking brain), we find ourselves in wise-mind mode (see the illustration on page 130). We can teach our children how to use both their logical and emotional thinking skills by modeling it ourselves and talking about our thought process out loud as we grapple between the two. By doing this, we assist them in cultivating more opportunities to access their wise-mind mode. Additionally, we also guide them in understanding the world and their position in it. Increasing our awareness of what frame of mind we're in helps us make better choices, build stronger relationships, and know ourselves better. Take a look at the activity box below on how to increase self-awareness.

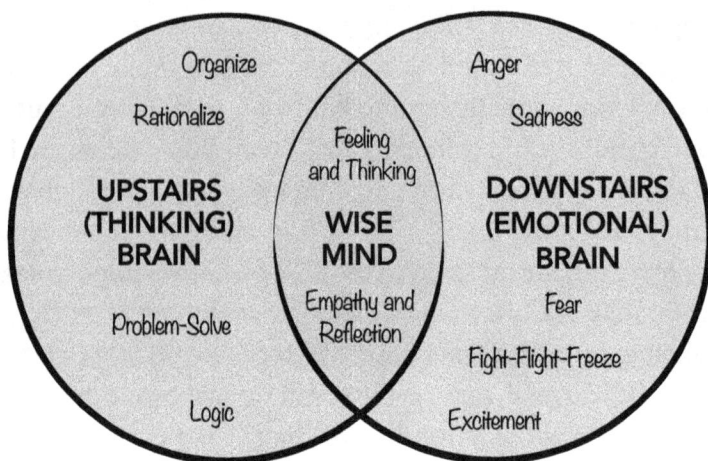

Organize
Rationalize
UPSTAIRS (THINKING) BRAIN
Problem-Solve
Logic

Feeling and Thinking
WISE MIND
Empathy and Reflection

Anger
Sadness
DOWNSTAIRS (EMOTIONAL) BRAIN
Fear
Fight-Flight-Freeze
Excitement

ACTIVITY BOX

Which mind do you rely on more when in a crisis? Your emotional mind (downstairs brain)—becoming very focused on feelings, becoming emotional yourself, over-empathizing with others, or getting cross/chaotic? Or your thinking mind (upstairs brain), where you might become solution-oriented, focused on rules/boundaries and facts, rely on words and logic?

Depending on your natural tendency to go toward emotions or logic, what do you need to help you bring the two minds together to be in a wise space when in crisis?

For example, could you use your emotional mind to connect with others through empathy, warmth, nonverbal body language, and your thinking mind to offer calm and reassuring words which can help make sense of what's happening and also consider problem-solving to help resolve the difficulty?

In the next week or so, try to notice which way your brain is pulled when in crisis. As you increase your awareness, use self-talk (talking through what you're noticing your brain is doing) to help bring back some balance.

Situations your child might face, their possible accompanying emotions, and the values these could signpost to

Situation	Emotion/Feeling	Value	Away moves	Toward moves	Exploration points
Rejection from a friendship group	Anger Fear Shame Hurt Sadness Guilt Confusion Disappointment	Loving/being loved Belonging Connection Community Kindness Friendship Loyalty	Withdrawing from others Saying/messaging unhelpful things Not trusting other people/friends	Reaching out to others Repairing relationship (saying sorry, resolving issues) Investing in good friendships	What do good friendships look like? How can you be a good friend? What other things can you do to help build belonging (join an activity group)? How can I/other adults help?
Failing an assignment	Shame Frustration Disappointment Embarrassment Guilt Worry	Achievement Ambition Pride Knowledge Learning Success Wisdom Self-discipline	Giving up Dropping the topic Not going to that lesson/school	Asking for help Doing more prep work Working out where you went wrong so you can learn from your mistake(s)	What are your aspirations/goals? What are your hopes for the future? What does success look like to you? How can I teach them the power of learning from failure? What structures/routines can support learning? How can I/other adults help?

Situation	Emotion/Feeling	Value	Away moves	Toward moves	Exploration points
Changing school	Fear Excitement	Belonging Inclusion Security Community Learning Career Growth	Avoiding going to school Not fully engaging with school or activities or new relationships	Being brave Investing in new relationships/ activities Opportunity for a new start	What are your hopes and dreams for school and the future? How would you like to feel at school? Are learning or social opportunities the priority? What can be done to support integration? How can I/other adults help?
Death of a loved one	Sadness Confusion Fear Hurt Guilt Anger	Loving/being loved Connection Care History/roots Forgiveness Legacy Safety Spirituality Health Vulnerability Peace	Withdrawing from others Not engaging in new relationships Blocking memories Getting rid of associated items	Reaching out to others Sharing grief and memories with others who cared about the person Investing in relationships Putting aside associated items until able to manage	What is/was the importance of the person in their life? How can I teach them about memories and legacy? How can I discuss the death of a loved one and how they can live on in you? How can I talk about how we let go? How can I encourage them to think about the power of love? What can we do to honor or commemorate that person—memory box, poem, letter? How can I/other adults help?

Situation	Emotion/Feeling	Value	Away moves	Toward moves	Exploration points
Not seeing a parent/parents separating	Sadness Fear Anger Guilt Hurt Insecurity Disappointment	Loving/being loved Connection Family Loyalty Security Care Commitment Belonging Harmony Friendship Honesty Truth Trust Respect Forgiveness	Withdrawing from others Saying or doing hurtful things Ruminating on who's to blame/revenge Black/white thinking: good/bad Taking too much responsibility Siding with one parent Seeing everything a parent does through a negative lens Shutting down communication	Reaching out for help Investing in family activities Sharing feelings constructively Repairing/rebuilding relationships Opportunity to know parents in a different way Staying close to siblings/other family members/friends	How do you view what a family is and what's the importance of that? How might this be changed or preserved? How can I explore things like commitment/loyalty as well as fears about loss of connection? How can I consider views on conflict and harmony? How can I explore routines and structures that might help make it easier? How can I provide balanced perspectives that acknowledge both sides of the story? How do I reckon with my own feelings as a parent? How can I/other adults help?

Situation	Emotion/Feeling	Value	Away moves	Toward moves	Exploration points
Adjusting to new siblings or a blended family	Fear Anger Envy Jealousy Insecurity Hurt	Loving/being loved Connection Fairness Uniqueness	Being in competition with/being unkind to/ withdrawing from parent Feeling unvalued Resenting others Behaving badly for attention	Investing in relationship with parent Trying to find ways to communicate fears Believing in love being infinite Embracing uniqueness Opportunity for new relationships/ friendship/fun	What is love? Can we love more than one person? What different things can we get from different relationships? How do we let others know what's important to us? What structures/routines can be introduced to support feeling fair/unique/special time? How can I help?
Losing a sports game	Anger Shame Sadness Disappointment Frustration Insecurity	Being the best Success Sportsmanship Teamwork Leadership Learning Belonging Fairness	Poor sportsmanship behaviors Not playing games in the future Giving up	Bringing team together to praise effort Exploring why and how the game was lost in order to build and practice skills to perform better next time Practicing good sportsmanship	How do we explore what was so difficult about losing the game (e.g., decisions made by the coach, player performance, bad luck, unfair decision/cheating)? How we do analyze these insights to reveal values around the game? What kind of behaviors would support these values going forward? How can I/other adults help?

SUMMARY

→   Painful or uncomfortable emotions are a necessary part of experiencing a full and meaningful life.

→   We cannot prevent our children experiencing painful emotions, but we can support them to make sense of these feelings and understand how they might tell us something about what's important to us.

→   Sitting with our children's feelings when they experience painful emotions gives us the opportunity to be in their world and honor their feelings.

→   It can be valuable to teach children the connection between their emotions and their developing values. By understanding why their feelings might hurt, they can learn to use their emotions to make wise decisions about their next steps.

→   Being more aware of our own feelings as parents can help ensure that we use both our downstairs (emotional) brains and upstairs (thinking) brains when we're supporting our children when they are distressed, and that we model "the wise mind."

PART 3
Anxiety
**How to stop it controlling
your child's life**

Chapter 7

Fear and the body

Every day, all of us experience events that trigger our fear or anxiety response. These can be things that are happening in our external world (e.g., work, school, money, health events) or our internal world (e.g., self-criticism, thoughts about the past and future). Anxiety is a natural part of life and can be our friend: it's something we all need to keep us safe, like stopping us from stepping in front of a bus. In fact, a small amount of anxiety can improve our performance. However, it can also be our foe. It can take up a lot of time and energy and stop us from doing the things that are most important to us, such as learning, maintaining relationships, and living a full and meaningful life.

During childhood, a third of children will experience difficulties with anxiety. It therefore makes sense that anxiety is one of the most common difficulties seen in mental health services. Many of the young people and families I meet through my work describe the disabling effect anxiety has on their lives. Parents often explain, with a degree of embarrassment, how much family life is impacted. Morning routines hampered by tummy aches and tears, the constant need for reassurance, and last-minute battles to get out of the house or car. Evenings where bedtimes become time-consuming and tension-inducing, because of worries about the next day and difficulties with sleep. The anxiety cycle is exhausting for both parents and children.

Do I need to worry about my child?

Throughout our children's growth and development, it's natural for them to experience worries and anxieties. As a parent, it can be difficult to know the difference between normal anxiety and anxiety that might require more support. I usually help parents work this out by finding out: (1) how much anxiety is getting in the way of their child doing things they would expect them to be able to do at their age; and (2) how long it has been going on.

Difficulties with anxiety can present in some children as a specific fear or worry that causes a problem in certain situations (e.g., a fear of dogs, insects, needles). Others may have more generalized anxiety that affects various areas of life (e.g., being away from parents, afraid of school, concerns about friendships). Typically, children who are likely to benefit from additional support are those who have been: (1) struggling with anxiety for a long time; and (2) finding anxiety is getting in the way of doing a range of things, like going to school and engaging in social activities. They are also the ones who will especially benefit from the tools in this book. However, as anxiety is such a universal emotion, these chapters will be helpful for all parents and children.

What does anxiety look like in a child?

Whether your child's fears and anxiety are new or old, occasional or constant, three main things happen while experiencing anxiety:

1. The body's stress system is activated, which causes biological changes in the body. These are unpleasant physical sensations, such as tummy aches and a racing heartbeat.

2. Thoughts tend to be focused on the negative and your child may find themselves worrying about the past, present, or future.

3. Your child might avoid things, seek out reassurance, or do things that will reduce the likelihood of the feared thing happening.

The table below illustrates how anxiety in these three areas might present on a day-to-day basis for your child. Circle the things that may apply to your child.

Physical sensations	Thoughts	Actions
Difficulties in concentration	"What if . . ." thoughts about the future often focused on the worst-case scenario	Avoiding feared situations (this can then grow to more situations)
Complaining of physical ailments (stomach pains, feeling sick, fatigue, shortness of breath, nausea, headaches, feeling shaky)	All-or-nothing thinking	Asking for reassurance from others
	Blaming self	Having routines or ways of doing things to help them feel safe
	Should/must thoughts	
	Discounting the positive	Difficulties with friendships
Reductions in sleep quality	Only paying attention to the negative	
Difficulties with digestion (loss of appetite, urges to go to the toilet, constipation)	Having high expectations of self	Spending more time with adults at home and school
	Blowing things out of proportion	
	Nightmares	

Some young people, especially teenagers, may be working hard to hide their feelings and worries. Most adolescents I meet with describe feeling ashamed of these feelings and not wanting to create more distress in their parents by sharing their anxieties. With older children, struggles with anxiety may present as being irritable and moody, enjoying things less, withdrawing from regular activities (e.g., going to school, meeting up with friends), becoming more easily upset, and needing more reassurance. Responding to these behaviors with kindness and curiosity is likely to be most helpful for your teenager, as their anxiety about you judging them will be high.

For younger children, anxiety can be masked by difficulties with behavior, anger outbursts, and temper tantrums. The next three chapters explain what anxiety is and guide you on what to do when your child's body, thoughts, and actions are affected by anxiety. Cognitive Behavioral Therapy (CBT) principles are woven into the text.

Why might my child struggle with anxiety?

There is unlikely to be a single reason your child might struggle with anxiety. Instead, research suggests the causes are multilayered and involve a combination of biological and environmental influences.[35] Below is a list of things that make children more vulnerable to difficulties with anxiety: see if any apply to your child.

* **Inherited factors:** Does a parent of your child have an anxiety disorder?

* **Temperament:** When your child was younger, did they have an inhibited temperament (quiet, not revealing thoughts/feelings)? Do they avoid or respond to new situations/people with reluctance or fear? Does your child interpret ambiguous information negatively (tend to predict the worst-case scenario, assume the worst)?

* **Environment:** Has your child had stressful life experiences? Has your child experienced emotional neglect or a negative or highly critical relationship with a caregiver?

* **Parenting:** Has your child consistently experienced their parent/s: (1) behaving anxiously, (2) presenting information to them negatively, (3) being overly involved with their activities and routines, and/or (4) discouraging independence?

If you feel a number of these apply to your child, the good news is that the information throughout this book will support the building of protective environmental and parenting factors, which will help build up your child's resilience in this area and protect them against these vulnerabilities.

A note on what's important

The worries that keep us awake at night are likely to be linked to the things that matter to us most (e.g., our children being healthy and happy, work, income, our own health, and our close and social relationships). They are also often influenced by past events that have caused us pain or fear. This is the same for our children. I've met with countless young people whose anxiety is affecting them at school, participating in activities with friends and taking part in family life. For some, this is triggered by a negative experience that has put these essential things in jeopardy. When I ask what's most important to them, young people tell me "doing well with my studies," "having good friends," and/or "being close to my family." At this point, we're able to acknowledge that the anxiety is not helping protect the things they care most about, but is instead putting these things at risk.

A useful way to teach your child how to take back control is by helping them realize that their anxiety isn't always helping them, and how it can become a hindrance. In my experience, showing the young person how anxiety is getting in the way of what's important to them is often the biggest catalyst to giving them the strength and motivation to stand up to it. With kind curiosity, you can create a safe space to have this discussion with your child (use the communication tips in chapter 13 to help you with this).

Young people I've supported in managing anxiety are often able to reframe some of the characteristics of anxiety as being helpful in enabling them to have the energy to be conscientious, caring individuals who are likely to work hard at making a contribution to relationships and in the workplace. In fact, we may find that we need some anxiety to help give us the energy to get things done. The tools in these chapters help ensure that anxiety stays a useful friend, rather than becoming an unhelpful enemy.

> ☁ **Reflection Box**
>
> Think about your child and answer these questions:
>
> 1. What is your child **most anxious** about right now?
> 2. What situations **trigger** anxious feelings in your child?
> 3. What other **emotions** does their anxiety connect to (e.g., feeling powerless, feeling not good enough, feeling unloved or unlovable)?
> 4. What earlier experiences may be influencing this?
> 5. Explore what's **most important** to your child right now. How does this explain their anxious feelings?
> 6. How is anxiety **moving them away** from what's important to them?
> 7. What **strengths** does your child bring to help them stand up to anxiety and move toward what's most important to them (e.g., humor, tenacity, loyalty, caring about others, energy/enthusiasm)?

What happens in the body?

Understanding what happens in our bodies when experiencing fear or anxiety is the first step to helping our children make sense of their feelings and appropriately reducing the intensity and frequency of them. This section will provide you with the tools to do this.

Introducing the stress system: Defense and recover

The brain has successfully evolved over millions of years to protect us from danger. It has developed a stress system that helps defend the body against harm (the sympathetic nervous system, which I'll refer to here as the stress response). It's essentially an alarm system that automatically: (1) tells us we're in danger; and (2) gets us out of danger as quickly as possible. Think of a caveman seeing a saber-toothed tiger: he needs to either run or fight to not be killed. The quicker and stronger the alert system to danger, the more likely the caveman is to survive.

To counterbalance the alert system, the caveman needs to make sure he does not waste energy unnecessarily, so he needs a good repair or restoration system to help him conserve and replenish his energy levels (the parasympathetic nervous system, which I'll refer to as the relaxation response). Both the stress response and the relaxation response happen in the brain and body without conscious control; they are automatic. To survive, all living things need their stress response and their relaxation response to work well together.

Stress response: Fight or flight

The stress response is the body's alert system to get out of danger. When we experience a stressful event, the stress response acts. The "event" could be something we see, hear, smell, taste, touch, or imagine that we perceive could do us harm. The part of the brain linked to survival and emotional processing (the amygdala) sends a distress signal to the part of our brain in control of the nervous system (hypothalamus). The hypothalamus sends a message through the nervous system to our adrenal glands, which then release a hormone called adrenaline into the bloodstream. This shot of adrenaline fires up the body ready for action. The heart rate increases and the blood in the body gets diverted to the muscles, away from the digestive areas (which is why the sensation of feeling sick, butterflies in the tummy, or needing to go to the toilet is felt). You breathe quicker, as your heart and muscles need more oxygen. Your muscles may tremble or shake and your arm hair might stand up to help you cool down quickly. Extra oxygen is sent to the brain, which may give tunnel vision to increase alertness, so you pay attention to the threat right in front of you. Everything is designed to provide the body with a short blast of energy to help you be as fast as possible to escape the dangerous situation (fight-flight).

This all happens in a nanosecond, before you're able to even process what you've seen, heard, or felt to create the alert. At this point, after the initial injection of adrenaline decreases, if danger is still perceived, the hypothalamus will send another signal to keep the stress response active. This produces cortisol, a hormone that keeps the body fired up in a state of fight-flight so that it can get out of danger. To be effective, the feelings in the body have to be as strong and as unpleasant as possible, so they can't be ignored and action is taken.

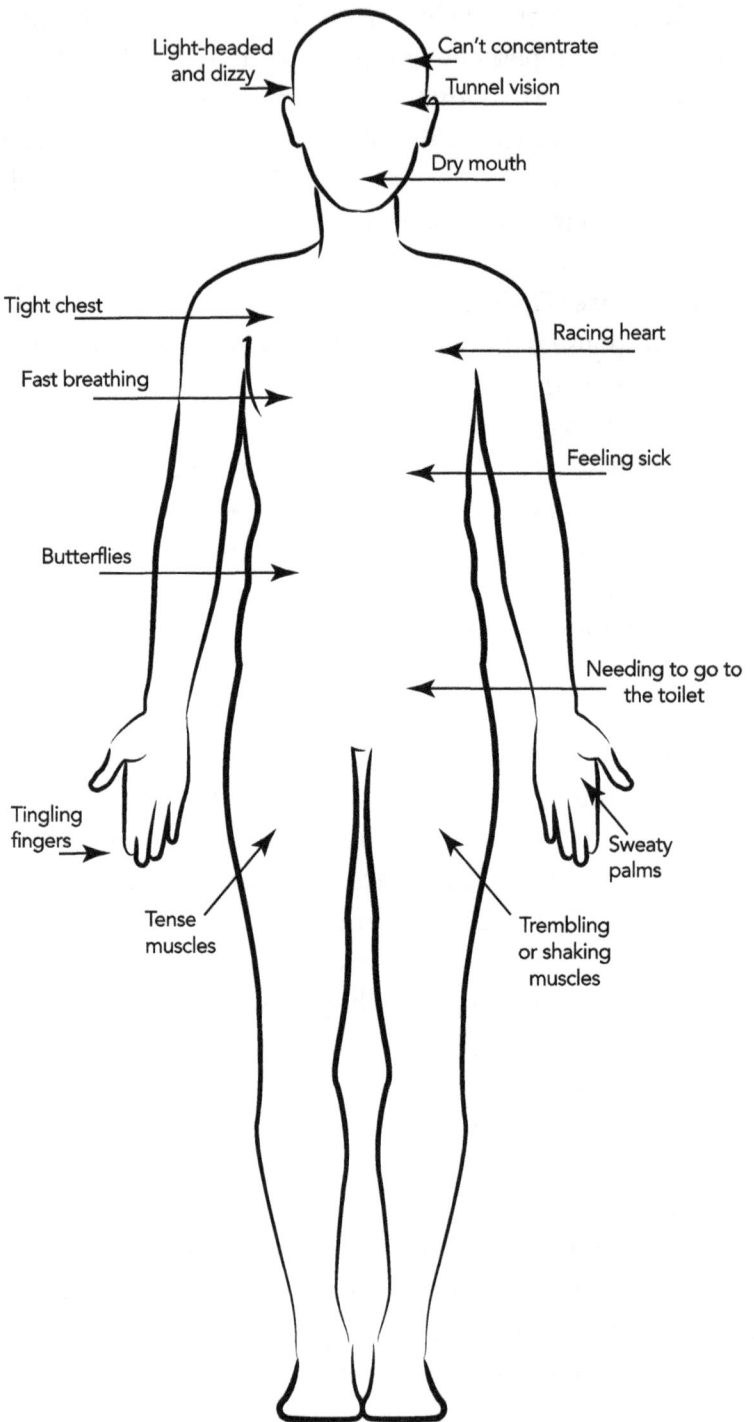

Light-headed and dizzy

Can't concentrate

Tunnel vision

Dry mouth

Tight chest

Racing heart

Fast breathing

Feeling sick

Butterflies

Needing to go to the toilet

Tingling fingers

Sweaty palms

Tense muscles

Trembling or shaking muscles

ACTIVITY BOX

Do this on your own

Think of the last time you felt afraid or anxious, then take a look at the picture on the facing page. What are some of the physical feelings you experienced? Now, think about your child. What are some of the physical sensations they complain of when feeling anxious or worried?

Do this with your child

Explain the fight-flight response to your child using the worksheet in the resource pack. Work out together how it affects their body. Sometimes children can confuse the feelings in their bodies as a sign of illness.

Fact Box

The chemistry behind breathing

Breathing is essential to life. It's an automatic process controlled by the brain. Most of the time we do not need to think about it. As we breathe, air is inhaled into our lungs and oxygen from this air enters our blood. At the same time, carbon dioxide, the waste product of breathing, moves from our blood into our lungs and is breathed out.

Our respiratory rate is linked to our body's energy requirements. When we exercise, we need to breathe more quickly so our body can take in more oxygen and expel more carbon dioxide. When we experience fight-flight, the adrenaline tells our body to breathe faster in preparation for physical activity. If we breathe faster, but aren't physically active, our muscles do not use up the extra oxygen in our blood. This creates an imbalance in the pH of our blood (respiratory alkalosis) and a drop in concentration of carbon dioxide, which constricts blood vessels and leads to us feeling light-headed, tingly in our fingers and toes, clammy and sweaty. While typically unpleasant for most people, it's not dangerous. You can help return your blood to a balanced state by slowing down your breathing or doing some physical activity, which will see off these sensations.

Will I faint?

These feelings can make a child worry they might faint. But fainting is very unlikely when experiencing anxious breathing. Fainting is typically linked to a drop in blood pressure and a reduction in oxygen to the brain. With anxious breathing, your blood pressure and oxygen levels are more likely to go up than down.

The relaxation response

In order to survive we not only need to escape danger, but we also need to conserve energy. The relaxation response complements the stress response. It controls the body's ability to relax by allowing it to rest (lower heart and breathing rate) and digest (ensure the body is processing food efficiently). The relaxation response relies on the vagus nerve communicating with the heart, the lungs and the digestive system to help it work most efficiently at conserving energy. It needs to kick in during or after a stressful event to help the body calm down and recover from being stressed. If the caveman stayed permanently stressed, he wouldn't be able to rest, sleep and eat, and would die from exhaustion.

When our children are very young, they rely on us to help keep their bodies safe. From when they are just babies, their stress response is already working to alert us, as parents, to protect them when things are not right. We then respond by reassuring them that they are safe, and soothing them, so their relaxation response kicks in, they stop being distressed and are able to settle. Think of a toddler scared by a firework's big bang and their parent helping to trigger their relaxation response by picking them up and soothing them. Through using their voice and touch, the child will now understand that the firework is not something that's going to hurt them, but is instead a pretty thing to appreciate. Some children may continue to rely on their parents or other adults to soothe them and activate the relaxation response and might require more reassurance. As they get older, our children need to learn to listen to their stress response and build the strength of their relaxation response. This will give them the skills to manage stress and stay safe.

When things get out of balance

In an ideal world, our stress response and relaxation response are well balanced. If we experienced a near-miss with a saber-toothed tiger, we would return to our cave (place of safety), tell our community about the incident and our relaxation response would kick in, enabling us to settle to eat and sleep, thus repairing our body from the exertion of escaping and recovering.

The problem with a stress system that has taken millions of years to evolve is that it has not adapted to modern-day stressors. We're exposed to many more constant pressures than the caveman, meaning our stress response is triggered more and we have less time to support the relaxation response. Even escaping is proving difficult, with smart-phones bringing some of the stress-inducing pressures into our safest places. This is particularly problematic as the stress response reacts the same to non-dangerous and imagined events as real or physically dangerous events, meaning even our thoughts can trigger the stress response (see the next chapter for more on this).

Many children experience one-off high-stress events, which can increase their anxiety, such as the death of a loved one. Others might experience chronic stressors that are keeping their stress response stuck "on." These young people may find themselves also experiencing low mood as their stress symptoms go into shutdown mode to cope with the constant stress.

For many young people, the situations they find themselves in when they are overwhelmed by anxious feelings in their body are not physically dangerous. They might be taking an exam, speaking in class, or going to a sleepover at a friend's house. The challenge is that these things are common and repeated on a daily basis (chronic), meaning our children's stress response is repeatedly being triggered, often unnecessarily. If our child's stress response is easily activated and they have limited opportunities for their relaxation response to be activated we may see this leads to our children struggling with sleeping, eating, concentration, and constantly being on edge and looking out for danger.

ACTIVITY BOX

Anxiety alerts your body to danger—much like a smoke alarm alerts you to a fire. However, sometimes a smoke alarm will go off and alert us when there is no fire (e.g., when cooking). Similarly, our bodies can cause us to feel anxious when there is nothing to be afraid of. Some children's alarms are more sensitive (for the reasons described earlier).

List the things that you think trigger your child's smoke alarm under two headings: non-physically dangerous and physically dangerous. Highlight the worries that are imagined. Which column is bigger for your child? How regularly is your child exposed to situations that trigger their alarm? What does your child rely on to switch off their smoke alarm?

Although the stress and relaxation responses are automatic, we can support them to stay in balance by: (1) being more aware of stressors and how they affect our body and (2) providing more opportunities for rest and recovery. Many everyday tasks may feel like stressors to your child, but it's important that they do not stop doing these activities, as this can cause the anxiety to grow and will not equip them to manage those stressors. Instead, we need to teach our children (and ourselves) to actively do more things that support the relaxation response, especially when we know we're experiencing more stressors. Some of these unnecessary stressors we can reduce for our child (e.g., exposure to conflict), but many stressors are unavoidable.

Research tells us there are a number of things that will typically trigger the stress response and a number of alternatives that will trigger the relaxation response.[36] This seesaw illustration explains this further.

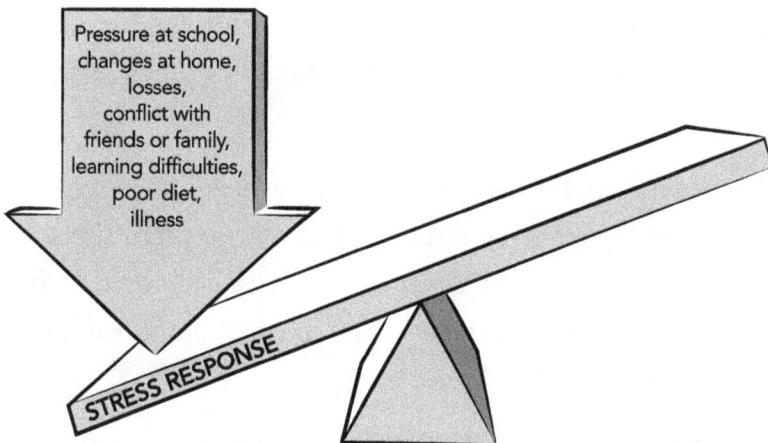

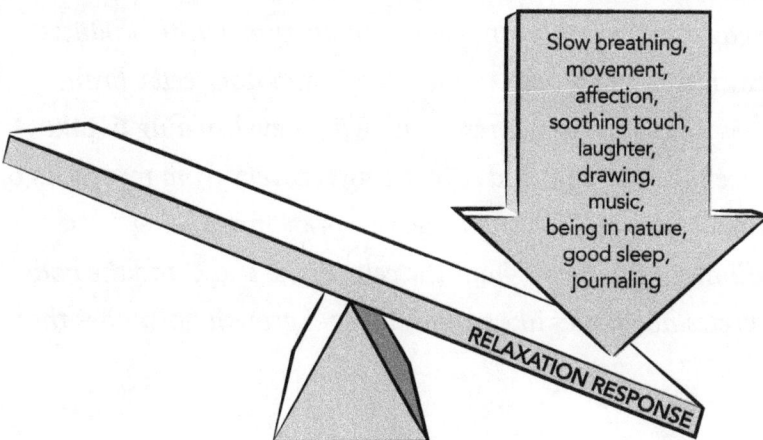

Pressure at school, changes at home, losses, conflict with friends or family, learning difficulties, poor diet, illness

STRESS RESPONSE

Slow breathing, movement, affection, soothing touch, laughter, drawing, music, being in nature, good sleep, journaling

RELAXATION RESPONSE

Fact Box

How sleep is affected by the stress/relaxation response balance

It's amazing to think that all living things have biological rhythms that are synchronized with the earth's movement around the sun. This built-in 24-hour clock in humans promotes being awake during the day and sleep at night (circadian rhythms). Again, this goes back to cavemen times. It's safer to sleep at night and be active during the day. Our circadian rhythm is reset each day when our eyes are exposed to morning light.

The circadian rhythm works in harmony with our stress response. In the morning, our stress response produces enough cortisol to increase our energy levels to help get us started and active. In the evening it deactivates the production of cortisol, as the body needs to move into the rest-and-digest zone.

Kasia Kozlowska and colleagues in their summary of the research describe how during the night while sleeping the body engages in an important clean-up function: waste products drain from the brain's immune-inflammatory cells, brain nerve cells shrink and reset (allowing new learning to take place the next day, and supporting recovery from memories of difficult events), the vagus nerve works on reducing inflammation throughout the cells in the body, and the body secretes hormones like melatonin and growth hormones that are fundamental for cell repair. Pain thresholds are reset. Lack of sleep leads to increased sensitivity to pain. During sleep, we fast (don't eat), which means our bodies also are able to focus on digestion and good gut health.

The harmony of the stress response and the circadian rhythm is important to health and wellbeing. Disruption in one area can lead to disruption in another, which is why disrupted sleep because of jet lag (traveling across time zones), shift work (working through the night), and experiences that create chronic stress have an impact on physical and mental health.

Sleep difficulties are commonly associated with anxiety, depression, and ADHD. For young people struggling with anxiety, research shows that worrying about school the night before interferes with going to sleep (which is why, quite often, once it's the weekend or holidays, sleep will improve). If children are worrying, whether they are experiencing adversity or not (as we will see in chapter 8), this triggers the stress response. This increases cortisol and disrupts the circadian rhythm, making it hard to go to sleep. Breathing exercises (page 155) and learning to manage worries better (page 171) are well-established ways to improve sleep by helping deactivate the stress response. Sleep interventions can help a young person learn techniques to significantly reduce the time it takes to fall asleep, reducing feelings of anxiety and low mood (see page 219 for top tips on improving sleep).

What are the ways we can build stronger relaxation responses in our children?

The power of breathing

The most effective way to activate our relaxation response and deactivate our stress response (fight-flight) is by controlling our breathing. When we're relaxed, at rest, adults breathe around six breaths per minute, and children/adolescents breathe around seven per minute. When we're afraid or anxious, we breathe more quickly, perhaps up to fifty breaths per minute, which increases our stress response and drives unpleasant fight-flight physical symptoms. Unlike other parts of our body, which we cannot consciously control, we're able to consciously control our breathing. If our breath is slow, it's impossible for our heart rate to stay high and our stress response to stay active. Slowing our breathing triggers the relaxation response, which signals to the rest of our body we're not in danger. It also decreases the experience of pain and increases a sense of wellbeing.[37] Therefore, learning to control breathing is one of the best ways to regain control of the body when experiencing stress.

There are lots of breathing exercises you can teach your children and phone apps to support this (refer to page 308). The key principles are: (1) slowing down the out-breath and breathing in more deeply (getting a good rhythm, using the diaphragm); and (2) moving away from over-focus on the fight-flight physical sensations. When introducing these to your child, do the exercises with them so they can practice getting the hang of it with you as their guide. Providing feedback to help them get the technique right is critical to enabling them to improve. Encourage them to build in daily practice of the exercises (see the practice activity box on page 160).

ACTIVITY BOX

Find a comfortable place to sit where you will be undisturbed, and turn off or remove distractions (phone, tablet, TV, etc.)

Deep breathing

1. Breathe in for four counts (try to inhale deeply so that the belly rounds out) and out for eight (say, "In, two, three, four. Out two, three, four, five, six, seven, eight" to help your child get the rhythm).

2. Repeat at least ten times.

3. Ask your child to count in their head while they do it. Counting helps calm the fight-flight response.

You may notice that when your child does this, they seem like they are running out of breath as they get to six, seven, eight. Helping them learn to breathe in deeply to the bottom of their lungs so that their belly expands will encourage them to have enough air to have a steady breath out. They will need to practice so it becomes less forced. If your child is younger, do this while lying down and ask them to place a teddy on their tummy. The teddy should go up and down as their stomach expands and they fill their lungs with and release the air.

Finger breathing

Spread out your fingers on your non-dominant hand (left hand if you're right-handed, right hand if you're left-handed). Use your finger from your dominant hand to trace up the outside of your thumb (take a breath in until you get to the tip), and as your finger traces down the other side of your thumb, breathe out. Breathe in again as you trace your index finger to the tip; breathe out as you trace down to the base of your middle finger. Complete for the remainder of your fingers (five full breaths). Repeat as many times as is helpful.

Grounding exercise

This is helpful for young people to do in lessons or situations where movement is limited and is a good exercise to introduce them to mindfulness. It's discreet and only takes a brief amount of time. When practicing with your child, encourage them to speak aloud. When they practise at school or in other similar situations, they can speak in their head.

1. Ask your child to name five things they can see, four things they can feel, three things they can hear, two things they can smell, and one thing they can taste.

2. Encourage detailed descriptions. This helps them pay attention to something other than how stressed they are feeling.

3. Ask them to relax their muscles at the same time by getting them to pretend they are a floppy rag doll—easing the muscles will also help the relaxation response.

There are many exercises online and the apps recommended on page 308 you can try with your children. Every child is different, so trying out a few will help them find their preference.

Movement

Research tells us that regular exercise protects us against depression and anxiety.[38] There appear to be lots of ways in which it does this. One way is by helping the brain release neurochemicals that improve a sense of wellbeing (endorphins, serotonin), while at the same time supporting the body in building a tolerance for stress hormones like cortisol. This enables the body to learn to get used to some of the physiological sensations that we might associate with the fight-flight response and reduce sensitivity to these anxious feelings. Exercise also helps the brain make new neurons (neurogenesis) in the part of the brain that supports mood regulation, learning, and memory (hippocampus), which means exercise for all of us (particularly helpful as we get older) improves nerve-cell connections in the brain.[39]

Activities and sports that involve movement and synchrony are especially helpful for reducing the stress response (e.g., drumming, dance).[40] If exercise provides a good enough challenge, it also builds a sense of self-efficacy and mastery. Opportunities to connect with others while moving our bodies can contribute to its positive effects (e.g., team sports, going for a walk/run or to the gym with a friend). Supporting your child to engage in physical activity that is meaningful for them can be a real game-changer. Sometimes anxiety will be preventing your child from engaging in these activities (e.g., anxiety about attending a sports club). Use the tools in chapters 8 and 9 to encourage your child to engage in more movement and physical activity.

Consider how you might model this to your child by integrating more movement into your daily life. Remember, just getting up and dancing around your kitchen for a couple of minutes to some music you enjoy can be enough to help relieve your stress response!

Practical ways to encourage the relaxation response

For many children, coming home after school or other stimulating events can be a difficult transition and you may see challenging behaviors. Children (and parents, too) need time to move from the pressure of the day/activity, which has kept the stress response active, to supporting their relaxation response to kick in. Remember the stress response helps release energy, so sometimes it can be helpful in enabling us or our child to get things done throughout the day. Structuring in regular downtime after stressful activities encourages the relaxation response. Preventing the stress response from becoming chronically activated can help avoid "burnout." We might find it hard to switch off the stress response when we get home or move to another activity, leaving us or our child feeling on edge and easily distressed. The first step to breaking the cycle is to work out with your child what works for them to support their relaxation response (the seesaw illustration on page 151 highlights activities that support this).

ACTIVITY BOX

Draw out the routine of the day with your child. Identify the likely stressors of the day, and incorporate activities to help build the relaxation response, especially following stressful activities. Be as specific as possible and support your child to get the ball rolling. Don't forget about food and mood: include meals and snacks. Once they've done the routine a few times, they will be able to take the lead themselves (see the resource pack for a worksheet to help with this).

Lots of young people like going to their room and having quiet time with a favorite TV show, or a relaxing activity like artwork or being with a pet for a little while after returning from school/a stressful activity.

The power of practice

Young people often come back to me saying, "Breathing slowly and deeply doesn't work." When I explore this with them it becomes clear that they do not see it as a skill they need to get better at, but rather as something they should automatically be able to do. I explain to them that controlled breathing is a skill and how, through practice, they can discover it *does* work. When learning a new skill such as a sport or an instrument, it's true that practice makes perfect. Talented people are not born talented; they become brilliant through practice. The challenge with practice is that it's uncomfortable, as it requires doing something we're initially not very good at and trying to improve. Practice requires motivation and bravery to help us tolerate these uncomfortable feelings without giving up. It also requires discipline: we need to do it every day to really get better. When we make something a habit, it becomes automatic. Research shows that we need immediate and helpful feedback to improve our performance, so make sure to support your child when they're learning something new.

Three things to help with practice

1. *As with any good habit, incorporate it into your daily routine.* For example, like cleaning your teeth, you can build breathing exercises into the bedtime routine. This is doubly helpful as when we're struggling with anxiety, sleep can also be more difficult.

2. *Set yourself up for success.* Little and often is better than a lot once in a while. We all like the feeling of success, but we have to start with an achievable goal. If I were planning to run a marathon in nine months' time, I wouldn't start running twenty miles today. I would start with short runs that I could manage without injury or putting myself off, and then build up my strength and fitness by extending my runs. The same goes with breathing—start with three minutes a day, then move toward your final goal of eight minutes a day.

3. *Don't expect to be able to use your breathing or new relaxation response skills straight away in a high-stress situation.* Practice when you're less stressed, in a situation that means you can really concentrate on practicing. For example, if you played the piano and I asked you to perform a tricky piece of music in front of a huge audience immediately, you probably wouldn't be able to do it well. The stress would make it virtually impossible. But if I suggested that you practice said piece every day for a month, and at the end of the month you would perform in front of a hundred people, you would have a much better chance of doing well. In this same vein, it's important to practice breathing every day for three minutes when you're calm and feel safe. Before you know it, you'll be able to slow your breathing down in a more stressful situation.

Don't give up if it doesn't help straight away. These things take time to develop and grow, like any new skill or habit. By doing the activities in this book, you're taking your brain to the gym! Like any muscle, the brain grows in the way we exercise it. The more we practice these activities, the stronger the neural connections in our brains become and the more able we are to manage stress and anxiety.

ACTIVITY BOX

How to help your child to build in practice

* For younger children, build opportunities to practice deep breathing into daytime routines. At bedtime, support them with a breathing exercise by placing a teddy on their tummy so they can see their breath going in and out. Once you've been practicing this in a low-stress situation, you can then support them to use their breathing when you see the warning signs they are getting distressed. Do it together and regularly, so they get in the habit, and they will soon be able to do it on their own.

* For older children and adolescents, encourage collaborative conversations about how to build opportunities to practice (see chapter 13 for the best ways to set these conversations up for success). Support them to come up with ideas that fit in around their other routines. Be curious and encourage them to come up with the ideas themselves. Write the ideas down together, or make a schedule. See my top tips on using scaling (e.g., 0 to 10) in chapter 2, which will help young people notice the benefits of doing the exercises and provides concrete feedback on what difference it's making.

* External rewards can support getting new habits established. Younger children might be happy with a sticker chart. Older children might like to link pocket money or privileges to successful completion of this. Praise and verbal recognition and encouragement of your child using their breathing will all help.

CASE STUDY

Noah's Story (Part 1)

**We will follow Noah through this and the
next two chapters as he tries out some of the tools
I'm sharing with you to help him manage anxiety.**

Noah is a fourteen-year-old boy in Year Ten. He's struggling with getting to school in the mornings, spending less time with his friends and finding his sleep and home life is disrupted. His parents have noticed he's irritable and doesn't want to join in with social activities with the family. He's constantly asking Mom for reassurance that everything will be OK. Some mornings, Mom has said that he doesn't need to go to school because Noah has been feeling sick, shaky and tearful.

Noah explained how important doing well at school and having good friendships was. We were able to identify that his feelings of fear and anxiety were mostly about not performing well at school and not being accepted in his friendship group. Noah was able to see that missing school or not spending time with his friends outside of school because of feeling this fear was taking him away from what was important to him. Not only did it make his anxiety worse, but it also made him feel low.

Noah and his parents were really interested when we went through the body picture to work out where Noah was feeling the fight-flight response. Noah was able to explain it wasn't just feeling sick and tearful, but that his heart was beating faster; he felt shaky and sometimes a bit light-headed too. Not being able to concentrate or listen to what the teacher was saying was making this fight-flight response get bigger because he worried that he would pass out in the lesson or the teacher would ask him a question and he wouldn't be able to answer. Once Noah understood how his brain and body were working, we went through the "In for four, out for eight" breathing exercise together in the room.

After this first session, Noah started paying more attention to the early signs of what was happening in his body. Over the following weeks, he was able to: (a) identify the feeling was his fight-flight response warning him of danger; and (b) do something helpful to let his body know that he was not in danger. He started using grounding exercises in lessons when he noticed he was feeling anxious, which allowed him to stop over-focusing on how his body felt and helped his relaxation response to kick in. We talked about the value of movement and other ways of supporting the relaxation response, and Noah built in the habit of walking the dog with his mom after dinner. At bedtime, Noah practiced deep breathing after cleaning his teeth. He found it helped if he listened to calming sounds on his phone while doing this; the sound of rain helped him focus on his breathing and not on his anxious thoughts, which made sleeping easier.

Noah's parents rewarded him for doing his practice regularly with praise and money toward a new pair of sneakers he was saving for. The family was less focused on the negative physical feelings and more focused on the activities Noah could do to feel like he had some control over them, allowing him to build his tolerance for the fight-flight feeling. This resulted in it passing more quickly.

- -

SUMMARY

→   Anxiety is normal. Everyone gets worried and scared sometimes.

→   Anxiety can be helpful in dangerous situations and protects us with the stress response to get our bodies out of danger quickly (fight-flight).

→   Anxiety can sometimes take over and stop us doing what's important to us.

→   The stress response gives our body a strong feeling to run or fight. It's an unpleasant feeling that we want to get away from.

→   The stress response is triggered when we're in non-dangerous situations or when we're worried. This can be difficult if we're afraid of things that are not going to harm us and these things occur regularly.

→   Our relaxation response protects us from stress and helps our bodies rest and digest, as well as helping our bodies recover from stress.

→   Deep breathing, movement, and other calming activities help activate our relaxation response to counterbalance our stress response.

→   Regularly practicing relaxation activities can help us cope with high-stress moments and manage chronic stress more effectively.

Chapter 8

What to do about worry

I'm sitting in the emergency department at my local hospital with my seventeen-year-old son who has a broken hand. It's 3 a.m., we have been here since 10 p.m., and we have not yet seen a doctor. Thankfully, he is calm and not in too much pain. While we wait, I reflect on the particularly challenging week. I seem to be juggling a lot of balls in my role as a mom, employee, ex-wife, friend, and writer! Consequently, I've been worrying a lot. Thoughts play on a loop in my mind, getting stuck on the past, present, and future, often playing out worst-case scenarios: *What if my house sale falls through? What if the big decision I made at work is a disaster for my team? What if I can't afford my fuel bills this winter? What if my friend is let down by me not replying to their message? What if the kids' dad hurts himself on his motorbike trip? What if I don't have enough time to write my book?* These and many more thoughts and imagined situations have been rolling around in my mind. Ironically, not for one moment did I think, *What if one of my children breaks their hand?* And yet here I am, in the hospital, with my son with a broken hand!

I'm sure that many of you can relate to this story. Despite worrying, in life you'll always experience an event that takes you by surprise and you haven't felt forewarned of. Life is unpredictable. It comes with risks. We don't always make the right decisions and often we have very little control over future events that can have a big impact on us and those we love. If we couple the uncertainty of life with the amazing brain's ability to imagine all sorts of possibilities, then it makes sense that worry is a feature of most people's lives.

Like anxiety, worry isn't all bad; it can be protective and draw our attention to problems that need solving (e.g., concerns about completing a time-dependent project at work). But it can also be disabling, chewing up time and energy and sometimes feeding us misinformation about situations (e.g., worrying about the possibility of a loved one being in an accident). As mentioned in chapter 7, anxiety affects three main areas: (1) our bodies, (2) our thoughts, and (3) our actions. It's not just real-life situations that can trigger our physical response to stress: it's our thoughts, too.

> ### Reflection Box
>
> Close your eyes and picture an event that has been unpleasant, or one that you would fear happening. As you're having these thoughts, pay attention to what's happening in your body. It's likely that you'll be able to notice some of the physical signs of anxiety that we explored in chapter 7, such as butterflies in your tummy, an increase in heart rate and breathing and perhaps feeling hot or cold. This is your stress response being triggered by your brain remembering or imagining these events. Now think of a pleasant event. Picture the event in your mind. Hopefully you will notice these physical signs of anxiety fading.

Many children I work with describe how worry is stopping them from learning, taking new opportunities, and building confidence. Parents describe their concerns that worry is controlling their child and getting in the way of them living a full and meaningful life.

I teach children and their parents that there is an art to "successful worrying," and show them practical ways to manage worry. This way, they can maintain a balance—being aware of risks, but not letting them dominate our thoughts and our future. In this chapter, I'll share these tools to help:

1. Challenge unhelpful thoughts.

2. Problem-solve rather than worry.

3. Let worry go when difficulties are outside of your or your child's control.

Thoughts and feelings

Recent research has discovered that we have around 6,200 new thoughts a day.[41] That's on average about 6.5 new thoughts a minute. These thoughts can be triggered by things that are happening around us, or our own thoughts. It's no wonder our minds can feel very busy at times! (Interestingly, this research found those adults with higher neuroticism scores had noisier minds at rest, were more easily distracted by their thoughts and their thoughts were more likely to involve distressing emotions.)[42] Our thoughts are linked to our feelings. Therefore, as this stream of constant thoughts passes through our mind, it will affect our mood. For example, if I think about the fact it's approaching Friday night and I have something nice planned, I feel a sense of pleasure as I anticipate being happy and relaxed. Alternatively, on Sunday night when I think about work the next day, I'll likely have a pang of anxiety and dread about Monday morning and the demands it will bring; I may then go on to imagine some of these possible challenges, and in turn increase my feelings of anxiety and dread.

The challenge is (as described in chapter 7) that our brains are hardwired for survival, not happiness. We are therefore much more inclined to look for the negatives in something than the positives (negativity bias), as from an evolutionary point of view this is more likely to help keep us safe—a caveman walking around looking at the flowers and not keeping an eye out for a predator is at greater risk of being eaten. This means we're inclined to give greater significance to negative thoughts, which can pose a problem when we start to notice and become hyper-focused on these unwanted thoughts. They often get stuck on a loop (this is called rumination), trigger our physical stress response (see chapter 7), and leave us feeling distressed.

Our world: Thoughts, feelings, and actions

Our experience of the world is based on what information we pay attention to and how we perceive, interpret, and describe what's happening. Any one situation can be viewed differently by a range of people. Take, for example, a child's first day at a new school. When my son and daughter started a new school following our recent house move, my son felt excited and positive about his first day. My daughter, however, felt anxious and worried.

When I collected my son and daughter, in both instances, they described meeting new people, getting to know a new building, having new teachers and new topics and orienting to a new routine. My son shared the things he had noticed that he liked about the new school, some boys that he played football with at lunchtime who supported the same team as him, the basketball court, the fact he did pretty well in the end-of-year tests considering he had not studied the topics. He focused on what went well, the new opportunities, and he saw himself as having been liked by others. There were a few things that had not gone to plan (e.g., he forgot his gym clothes), but he did not overly dwell on these. He finished the day looking forward to the rest of the week.

My daughter, in contrast, focused on the things that she had paid most attention to. These were the new rules of high school (which she felt were stupid and controlling), how the lunchtime arrangements meant she couldn't see some of her friends and, therefore, in all probability she would lose these friendships, and how she was always going to be getting late marks because the school site was too big. She felt her math teacher was very strict and may not like her, so going forward she predicted the class was going to be a nightmare. Lastly, she had been put in the top set for English, "but only because everyone else is useless." She finished the day dreading the rest of the week.

Two important things to note about these experiences of a first day at school:

1. What my son and daughter paid attention to and what they ignored throughout the day influenced what **they thought**, what **they did**, and how **they felt** about themselves and others (illustrated below).
2. What my son and daughter did as a result of their thoughts and feelings influenced what others around them did in response.

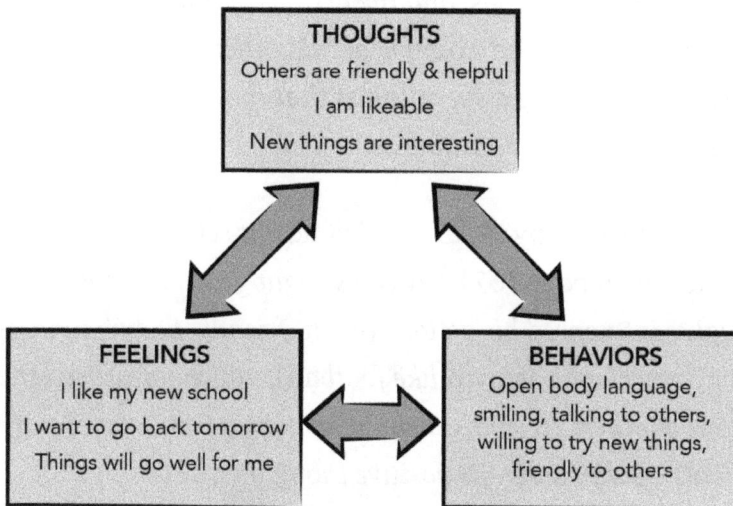

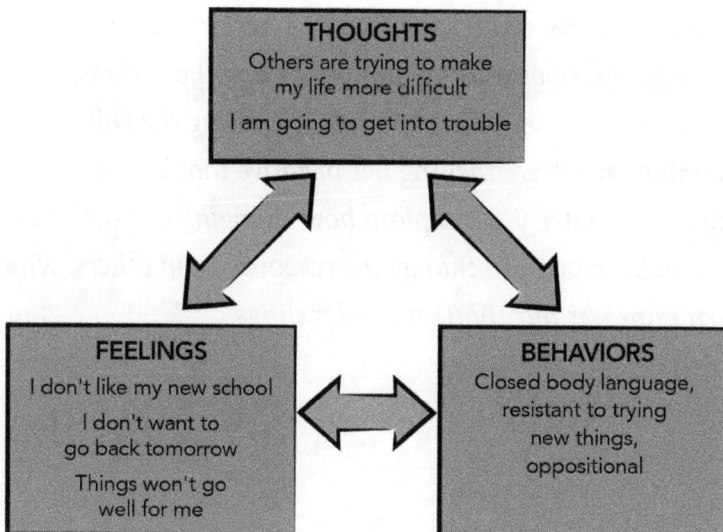

THOUGHTS
Others are friendly & helpful
I am likeable
New things are interesting

FEELINGS
I like my new school
I want to go back tomorrow
Things will go well for me

BEHAVIORS
Open body language, smiling, talking to others, willing to try new things, friendly to others

THOUGHTS
Others are trying to make my life more difficult
I am going to get into trouble

FEELINGS
I don't like my new school
I don't want to go back tomorrow
Things won't go well for me

BEHAVIORS
Closed body language, resistant to trying new things, oppositional

(see
illustration on page 167)

-☼- **Fact Box**

Self-fulfilling prophecy

*Research has found that our beliefs (thoughts) can predict
what happens next. Not because our thoughts are correct, but
because they affect what we expect, and in turn what we pay
attention to, our actions, and the actions of others.*[43] *The
placebo effect is a good example of this, whereby patients feel
better after receiving a sugar tablet that they believed was
medication to treat their illness.*

*In the example of my children's first day at school (see
illustration on page 167), my son's (light gray box) positive
thoughts influenced his actions (open, friendly body language,
doing activities he enjoyed like football), which influenced the
actions of others (friendly, helpful responses from school staff/
students), confirming his positive thoughts and feelings
(making them stronger). In contrast, my daughter's (dark
gray box) negative thoughts influenced her actions (closed
body language, oppositional approach) and the actions of
others (others warier of her, teachers imposing the rules),
confirming and strengthening her negative thoughts and
feelings. In chapter 9, I'll explain how changing our actions
alone can be enough to change the response from others, which
in turn improves our thoughts and feelings.*

As parents, our beliefs/worries about what to expect from or
for our children, or what they can manage, can influence: (1)
what we notice about them and their world and (2) our
actions. This can unintentionally reinforce our beliefs/worries.
For example, if I worry my child is not going to cope well at
their new school, I might fixate on the negative details of their
experiences in school. I may also try to protect them from
managing some of these problems themselves, reinforcing the
belief that they can't cope, and not giving them the opportunity
to learn through their own actions what they are capable of.

Unhelpful thinking styles

All of us will have thinking styles that can be helpful or unhelpful.
These are habits of the brain that aid us in processing and compre-
hending the world around us. In the above example, we can see some
of the unhelpful thinking styles that influenced my daughter's first day
at high school.

Looking at the Reflection Box on the next page, which types of
unhelpful thinking styles do you recognize? Do you notice yourself or
your child getting stuck in any of these types of thinking? Can you
make the link between these patterns of thinking styles and the feelings they trigger?

I've provided you with an example. See if you can write down your
own example of something you've thought in the last few weeks or
heard your child say that might fit under these headings. How do these
thoughts make you or your child feel? Some thoughts might include
more than one type of thinking.

☁ Reflection Box

All-or-nothing thinking

"I'm always going to be late for lessons."

Jumping to conclusions

"My teacher is strict; she doesn't like me." (Imagining we know what others are thinking.)

"I'm going to hate math lessons." (Predicting the future.)

Catastrophizing—blowing things out of proportion

"I'm not going to see all of my friends at lunchtime, so they are going to hate me, then I'll end up with no friends."

Minimizing—making something (which could be good) seem less significant

"I'm only in top set because everyone else is useless."

Discounting the good things

"It doesn't count that English went well; math was terrible."

Labeling

"I'm useless"; "School rules are stupid and controlling."

Blaming self

"It's my fault my friends couldn't find me at lunchtime."

The challenge with thoughts is that they often *feel* like facts. The strong feelings they create in us can convince us that they represent the truth or predict the future. Often, we assume that if we feel a certain way, what we think must be true. For example, if I think that Monday morning is going to be too difficult to cope with, I'll feel anxious, and this feeling will make me more certain that Monday is going to be too difficult to cope with. My thought has started to feel like a fact and takes on more power. In reality, Monday morning may be difficult, but I'm likely to be able to cope with it.

Train the brain

The beauty of the brain is that we can train it. Although our children are biologically programmed to notice the tough stuff and it's easy to fall into the habit of getting stuck in worry or negative thinking (especially if they've had difficult experiences), we can support them in breaking free from this cycle by teaching them positive and encouraging self-talk, sharing tools for problem-solving, and showing them how to let go.

Challenging worry myths

All of us have a view on the role and purpose of worrying. It might be that we believe that by worrying, we can prevent bad things happening. Some of the beliefs we have about worry can make it harder to give it up. It's important to be aware of this for you and your child, because when we challenge worry, we might discover that our child wants to hold onto it because he or she believes it has a value or a purpose. If we believe there are benefits to us worrying, how likely are we to give up worrying? Complete the worry myth activity below to explore which of these statements apply to you and/or your child.

ACTIVITY BOX

Have a look at these worry statements. Many of us have at least one that we believe in and some of us will have several. Go through each statement and consider, "Do I believe this? Does my child believe this?"

Worry statements
Worrying helps me cope with things.
If I keep worrying, bad things will not happen.
Worrying helps me solve problems.
If I worry, I'll be motivated to do things.
Worrying shows I care.
Worry helps me prepare for the worst.

It's important to dispel the worry statements above as myths—here's advice on how.

Worry helps me prepare for ...

It's not the act of *worrying* (repetitive thinking about a problem in a negative way) that helps prepare for something, but the act of *problem-solving* (solution-focused). We can support our child to get into the habit of noticing worry and making it productive by using the worry tree (see page 176) to address worries within their control through working out how to solve the problem. The challenge with believing worry always prepares you for the worst is that it leads your mind to focus on potential problems. This prevents you from experiencing the positives that are happening in your life and can contaminate these moments. As we explored earlier in the chapter, it can lead you to having expectations that influence your actions. By over-focusing on your worries, you could make them *more* likely to happen, not less.

If I worry, I'll be motivated to do things/ Worry shows I care

You may think that you need to worry to be motivated enough to get things done. Although some anxiety or worry is helpful to encourage us to take action, getting stuck with worry reduces effective action and often leads to a reduction in mood. Test this out by rating your mood (1–10, low to high) when you're worrying, compared to when you're not worrying. Here you'll see that your mood is likely to be lower when worrying more and will most likely reduce your productivity. Furthermore, worrying can diminish our ability to form connections with others, which can make it more challenging for us to show our care for others through actions.

If I keep worrying, bad things will not happen

Many children I work with have the misconception that worrying can prevent bad things from happening. Though this belief isn't logical, it's still influential because disproving it means stopping worrying and facing the possibility of the bad outcome, leading to increased anxiety in the short term. It's the same with negative and unhelpful thoughts. Rather than assuming the worry myth or negative thought is true, I help children become a detective by teaching them to investigate their thoughts, rather than simply believing them. This involves spending time searching for **evidence for** the worry belief or the negative thought and **evidence against** their worry belief or negative thought. (See the activity sheet in the resource pack if you would like to try this at home.) This technique can help your child approach a thought with more curiosity, rather than assuming it's 100 percent correct. It can also give them the opportunity to develop more balanced self-talk to counteract the negative energy a thought might be having.

Words of encouragement:
What we say to ourselves

Many of us worry about worry! In fact, a lot of the teenagers I meet with tell me how worried they are that their worrying thoughts mean they have a mental health problem. I explain it's normal to feel unsettled when we have uncertainty in our lives. Worry is what our minds have evolved to do to keep us safe. However, it's what we *do* with worry that matters. Do we use it to help us, or allow it to control us?

Some young people struggle to put words to their thoughts and feelings. Yet words are such a powerful way to define and frame our experiences. Using them constructively can support our brains in learning habits that improve our mood and reduce anxiety. I often ask young people to spot their negative thoughts and find key phrases they can write down to uplift them when their thoughts are becoming unhelpful. For example, instead of "I can't do this, I'm rubbish," reframe this as "I can do this with a bit of practice/help."

Demonstrating this habit to our children by doing it ourselves is the most valuable way to teach them. If we have negative, unhelpful thoughts and worries rumbling about our minds, we can counteract them with some kind, encouraging, and positive statements. This teaches our children that: (a) it's normal to have worries or negative thoughts and (b) there are ways we can help challenge them or not let them be so powerful. I have to force myself to do this all the time. My children will often hear me say things like:

"Give yourself a break, Beth, you might have forgotten to do that task, but think about all the other things you remembered today."

"I'm shouting again; it makes me feel like a terrible parent, but if I listen to that thought I'm going to get more upset. Sorry, kids—let's try again; what shall we have for dinner? We're all hungry and that means I'm more easily getting cross—let's make life easy tonight and have something quick for dinner."

I encourage young people and parents to practice talking to themselves like they would with a best friend. Say your feelings aloud in a way that makes sense to your children and gives them permission to notice difficult thoughts, providing self-support rather than self-criticism.

ACTIVITY BOX

Try this for yourself, so that when you support your child with the task, you understand and know how it works. Think of a phrase that often comes into your head when you're feeling worried or anxious, and write it down (e.g., "I can't do this. I don't want to give it a go; I'll mess it up").

Now, think of a phrase that encourages you to acknowledge the feeling/worry, but not let it control or dominate you. The only two rules are: it needs to be (a) realistic, and (b) kind, such as "I'm feeling anxious because I want to do a good job; that's OK. If I give it a go, I can be proud of myself whatever the outcome. I can do this."

Write this phrase down on paper and carry it around with you in your pocket or keep it on your phone. Read it regularly, especially when worries/negative thoughts show up.

The worry tree: Nobody solves a problem like . . .

Our children's worries are likely to be varied. They might feature things that they have some control over (e.g., "What if I fail my exams?") and other worries that they may have no control over (e.g., "What if my parent gets hurt in a car crash?"). It's valuable to help our children to distinguish between the two. Worry might help your child to identify a problem that needs solving, so rather than getting stuck with the worry, helping your child come up with an action plan to resolve the problem is a great life skill and builds psychological flexibility, crucial for adjusting to life's challenges and for wellbeing.

The worry tree[44] is a visual tool that you can share with your child when there is something that is bothering them (see illustration). It

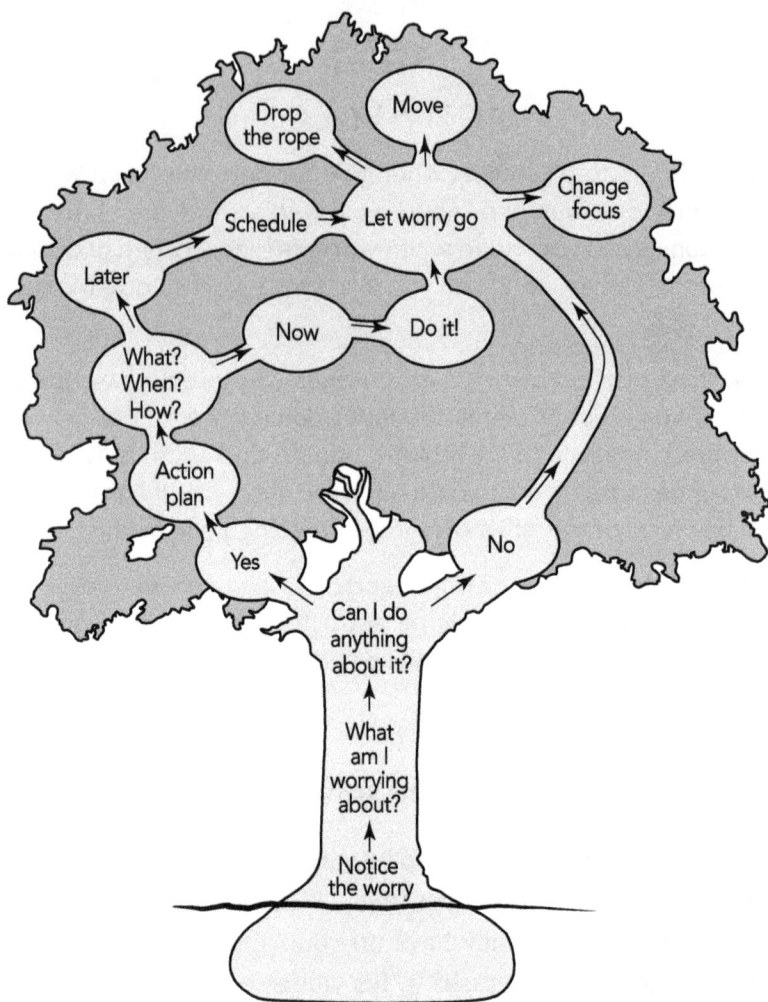

helps you both work out whether the worry is a problem or not. If it is, it guides them through the stages required to resolve the problem. If it isn't, it helps them identify that they need to let the worry go, and/ or change the focus of their attention. (The drop-the-rope exercise on page 181 gives you and them the tools to do this.)

Both the worry tree and the drop-the-rope exercise help your child build a strong connection between their upstairs and downstairs brain (see chapter 4) and triggers the relaxation response (see chapter 7).

As the stress response is designed to help us to take action, by problem-solving in this way, we're supporting the brain to feel the necessary action has taken place, so we can move toward feeling safe again.

To show you how to use the worry tree with your child, I'm going to describe how I used it with a student I worked with.

Remember Noah from chapter 7? He was struggling to go to school because of worries about his work and friends. Noah explained that he felt he was constantly worrying about everything. This was impacting on him wanting to go to school and spend time with his friends. It also meant that when he was at school or with his friends, he was constantly looking out for things that confirmed his worries were true. I asked Noah if we could look at one of his big worries and use the worry tree to help us work out what to do with it. Together, we drew it on a piece of paper and wrote down some ideas around it. By putting it on paper, this helped to make the worry seem less powerful.

1. *Notice the worry*
   First, I asked Noah to notice/pay attention to the details of the worry. In this situation, we thought about a particular worry that had been bothering him that week—something that kept popping into his mind and getting in the way of things.
   Noah explained he had a math mock exam in two weeks.

2. *Ask, "What am I worrying about?"*
   Noah explained math was a subject he found harder than his other lessons and he was worried he was going to fail the test, or, worse, be so anxious he might not be able to stay in the exam hall.

3. *Ask, "Can I do anything about it?"*
   Noah said that although he couldn't stop the exam going ahead, he could do something about doing badly and managing feeling anxious.

4. *Action plan*

Rather than jumping in with the solutions (I was tempted), I asked him to come up with as many different ideas as to what he could do, even if they seemed silly, to help him solve this problem. He explored ideas: not going to the exam, doing revision, going to the exam and cheating, speaking to his teacher for some extra practice papers, doing the breathing and grounding exercises he had learned in our previous session. We went through the pros and cons of each and Noah was then able to consider which was the best solution. When coming up with this, hold in mind what's important to your child. For Noah, this was doing well academically and feeling more confident with his friends. Therefore, not going to the exam, going and cheating, or leaving the exam early wouldn't be a good solution for Noah as it wouldn't help him get closer to what was most important to him.

5. *What? When? How?*

This is a crucial phase that often gets missed out when we're supporting our children in problem-solving. It's helpful to explore with them exactly what they are going to do, when they are going to do it and how. This enables them to troubleshoot problems that might prevent them completing their action plan, and it also makes the task more manageable and likely to be achieved. Remember, support them to come up with the ideas rather than coming up with the ideas yourself. Guide them if some of their ideas might be unrealistic, as setting reachable goals builds confidence and motivation.

Noah came up with the **what**: revision and practicing breathing/grounding exercises; and **when**: for forty-five minutes each night (he had suggested an hour, but we worked out together that forty-five minutes was more achievable), after dinner in his room (putting his phone on silent to avoid

distractions), doing his deep breathing (see page 155) for
three minutes before bed. During the day, he would complete
his grounding exercise at least once (see page 156). And for
the **how**: he would ask his teacher for additional practice
papers. At the weekend, Noah could connect with a friend
online and study together since his friend was also concerned
about the upcoming exam.

6. *Now?*
   We worked out what Noah could do immediately. I encouraged
   him to focus on completing these tasks then and there. He
   texted his friend and asked if they could meet online to revise
   over the weekend. He wrote in his school planner the topics he
   planned to cover each evening over the next two weeks.

7. *Later?*
   For the things Noah couldn't do immediately, we planned
   what he could do later and when he would do it. Noah had
   math first thing in the morning, so he put in his planner to
   speak to the teacher about practice papers. He also asked
   his mom to send an email to school that evening, so he
   was confident his teacher would be prepared to give him
   the papers the next day. Noah started the forty-five-minute
   revision session that evening, after dinner (he would ask his
   parents to try to have dinner at the same time most nights to
   help with keeping the routine), and he committed to his three-
   minute deep breathing and grounding exercise every day.

Noah appeared visibly relaxed after completing the exercise. I asked
him to spend the next week making sure he noticed when the worry
about his math mock exam came up. Rather than getting sucked into
the cycle of worry, he could kindly remind his brain, "I have a good
plan to deal with this problem; I can let the worry go."

The worry-meter

Helping your child put a number to the intensity of their feeling or worry can help them notice more objectively what they are experiencing. It also allows you to think collectively about practical ways to reduce the intensity of the feeling. At the beginning of the worry-tree exercise, I asked Noah, "How much are you worrying about your maths mock out of ten, with ten being all the time and zero being none of the time?" Noah said eight. After completing the worry-tree activity together, I asked him, "How much are you worrying about your maths mock out of ten?" He told me it was now a 6. This helped him see the benefit of doing the activity.

If completing the worry-tree exercise didn't help sufficiently, I could move to supporting Noah to complete the drop-the-rope exercise (more on this below). Alternatively, Noah could accept that, for a while, he might feel like an 8, but the feeling will pass and he can ride it out rather than getting caught up with it.

To help your child when they're feeling worried, you can use the worry-meter below. This tool will remind them of the various activities they can do to ease their worries. Having a worry toolkit enables young people to feel more in control of their worries and reminds them that they can choose how to respond to them. It's important to note that worry is a natural part of life, and we cannot eliminate it completely. Nonetheless, we can learn effective strategies to reduce our worry levels when they start to become overwhelming.

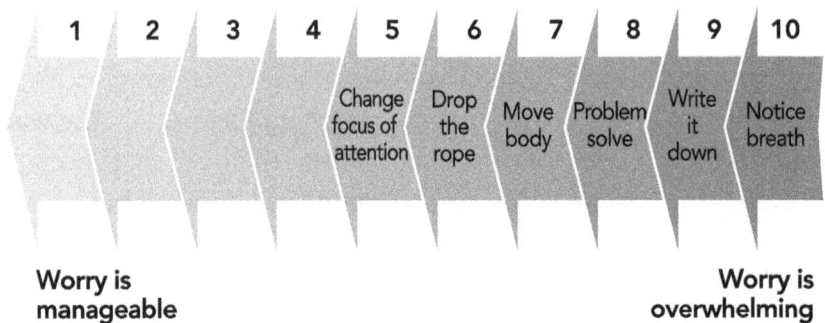

1	2	3	4	5	6	7	8	9	10
				Change focus of attention	Drop the rope	Move body	Problem solve	Write it down	Notice breath

Worry is manageable　　　　　　　　　　　　　　　**Worry is overwhelming**

Letting worry go: Drop the rope

Simply trying to stop or block worries or unhelpful thoughts does not work. If we do this we end up in a battle with the thoughts, using up energy, which leaves us feeling even more out of control. The challenge with focusing too much on positive thinking as a solution to negative thinking is that there are many times in life when we should naturally be feeling painful and difficult emotions (as described in part 2). Making space to feel these will enable us to cope better in the longer term. By processing the feelings, they won't keep coming back to get our attention.

I use an exercise from Acceptance and Commitment Therapy (ACT)[45] with children and young people which involves me taking one end of a length of rope and asking them to take the other. I tell them to imagine I'm a big worry monster and tell them to pull with all their might because in between us is a big, bottomless pit. They use all their energy up by pulling because they are sure that if they lose, they'll be pulled into the pit. But the harder they pull, the monster pulls harder. I ask them, "What's the best thing to do here?" Often a young person might say, "Pull harder." I'll reply, "Well, your mind will tell you to keep pulling, harder and harder. But the monster never seems to tire. You're still stuck. So, what's the best thing to do now?" At this point, the young person lets go. On dropping the rope, they realize their hands and legs are free—no longer stuck in the battle. By not getting caught up with the worry monster and accepting it remains present—the monster's not been pulled into the pit to never be seen again—the young person can use their energy to get on with doing something more helpful or rewarding, despite the worry monster still being present. At this point, the worry monster loses its power.

If you've completed the worry-tree exercise with your child and the worry is not within their control, try the drop-the-rope exercise with your child.

ACTIVITY BOX

Help your child to notice when they are caught up in their worries. When the brain is racing, it's hard to tell when you're getting drawn into a downward spiral.

1. Support your child to slow down their breathing and/or complete a grounding exercise (page 156) to help their bodies feel less hyperaroused.

2. Ask your child to pay attention to the feelings they are experiencing and encourage them to stay in the present and not fixate on the past or future. Using drawing or writing to express their thoughts can be helpful and there are journaling tools for children of all ages, which you can buy to support this activity. Writing about emotional events, either positive or negative, is associated with health and wellbeing benefits.[46]

3. These activities are not about stopping the brain from having certain thoughts. Instead, they are about choosing whether to get caught up with them. Thoughts can come and go. With practice, your child can choose not to pay unnecessary attention to them.

4. Distancing creates space between the thought and the person. Take the power out of the thought by introducing some fun. If your child says the thought in a funny voice, this can help the thought lose its potency. Capturing the thought on paper or talking to someone about the thought can reduce the intensity of the worry.

5. Movement is one of the most powerful ways to reconnect with your body and the space around you. Moving to a different space, trying a different activity, or walking around and observing your environment can transfer the focus of attention from your thoughts to the world around you. This can be especially powerful at night when children are more likely to get stuck with worries. Listening to music, soothing sounds, or

white noise can shift the focus of attention, and getting out of bed to move around (even if it's to do a boring activity) can help prevent further distress.

How else can we support our young people to drop the rope?

If our children are caught up in worry, it's likely to be about something that is important to them. It's vital to help our children recognize that their emotions are signposts to what matters to them. For example, Noah was worried about the things he valued most—doing well at school academically and having good friendships. If something difficult, painful, or confusing happens to any of us it can sometimes lead to further confusion or distress. Having others help us make sense of this can be transformational.

As parents, we're in a good place to support our child to do more activities that are in line with what they really care about and what's good for their wellbeing (the Wellbeing Abacus can help). Look at their weekly routines to explore how much they are engaging in these things. Build in opportunities for your child to have access to more meaningful activities (e.g., playing football, having a friend over to play, spending more time with you).

Hold in mind that difficulties in children's wellbeing occur when they are not finding satisfaction in activities that are important to them. So, your child might be doing things they value, but they may struggle with these things because of the need to learn new skills in this area (e.g., a child who wants to spend more time with friends, but struggles with their social skills, so time with friends is difficult). Parents can use their child's initial worry to explore further how their child might need more support to build skills in a particular area (e.g., "I'm really worried about going to this party" can lead to rehearsing the things that the child might need to do to help the party go well for them).

This approach helps to build confidence and provides more chances to successfully manage uncertain situations. Such experiences provide your child with a sense of hope that they "can do this" with the right help. This creates a healthy foundation to work from, rather than them not doing things because of a fear of failure or the unknown. Acknowledging difficult feelings and facing challenges despite these is how our children learn to be brave and do things that matter to them. Think, "I really want to go to the party and I'm anxious" rather than "I'm anxious so I can't go to the party."

We cannot protect our children from all that life might bring. Equipping them with skills to embrace uncertainty rather than live in its shadow is a powerful gift to offer your child. In the next chapter, we will explore how we can support our children to be brave in the face of the things that make them feel anxious. But before we do, here's a simple gratitude exercise you can practice with your child.

ACTIVITY BOX

Research tells us that gratitude (an attitude of thankfulness) is strongly related to wellbeing, including reductions in stress and improvements in sleep, coping, and relationships.[47] Scientists have found that the simple exercise below increases gratitude and improves wellbeing. Give it a go—you should see the benefits within two weeks.

* Every night, before bed, write down three to five things you're grateful for.

* For younger children, as part of their bedtime routine, you can ask them to name three things they are grateful for (or happy about).

* For older children and adolescents, explain that scientists have found that writing down just three things a day you're grateful for (or happy about) helps improve wellbeing. Encourage them to

keep these lists in a notebook or on their phone. There are lots of apps to help (e.g., Three Good Things).

✻ To build the habit into family life, you could ask each of your family members at mealtimes: "What has happened today that you're grateful for?" rather than "How has your day been?"

✻ Appreciating the things we usually take for granted is the key to this exercise, so find simple things to make the task easier (e.g., "I'm grateful I have food to eat, a comfy bed to sleep in, a mom who loves me, eyes to see, a friend who makes me laugh").

✻ Daily journaling[48] (writing thoughts and feelings linked to what's happening in your everyday life) is another practical way research suggests improves wellbeing and health. The act of keeping a diary helps encourage gratitude; it also provides an opportunity to become more self-aware and express difficult feelings. Giving meaning to difficult experiences through this process can support resilience. Again, doing this activity yourself as well as encouraging your child to get into this habit (through pen and paper or a journaling app) is a simple, practical tool to consolidate the skills you've learned about in this chapter.

SUMMARY

→ Worry is a natural part of being human. Like the stress response, we have evolved to notice the tough stuff to keep us safe from danger.

→ Our thoughts are powerful. They influence what we notice in our world, how we make sense of it, what we feel, and what we do.

→ Our stress response is triggered by our thoughts. Getting stuck with unhelpful thoughts can lead to worry, dominating our time and having a negative influence on the outcome of events.

→ Children may believe that worry helps protect them from bad things happening. We need to support them to find opportunities to:

• use encouraging self-talk to shift the tendency to focus on the negative;

- problem-solve when they face worries they can do something about;

- let go when they don't have control over things they are worrying about.

→ Unexpected events in life contribute to worry. If we support children in believing they have the resources to cope, they are more likely to experience the world with a sense of curiosity, confidence, and hope, providing more opportunities to grow and learn.

→ Simple activities, like listing three things you're happy about, or grateful for, every day, can improve wellbeing and mindset by helping you focus on the positive things you already have, and may often take for granted.

Chapter 9

Acts of courage

Many years ago, when I was in my twenties, I had a frightening experience flying back to the UK from New York. The turbulence was so bad that I spent eight hours fearing I would never make it back to solid ground. I swore, "If I survive this flight, I'll never fly again!"

I made it safely home, but for the following five years, I refused to fly. I was sure that if I did fly, I would either: (1) die in a plane crash or (2) even if the flight was uneventful, I wouldn't be able to cope with the anxiety I'd felt on the New York flight again. Although this did not impact my life on a daily basis, it meant that I turned down opportunities to travel for work to attend events, such as a conference abroad I had been asked to present at. Any holiday I took involved driving rather than flying! When I contemplated flying, I was filled with a wave of dread so strong that I was convinced that the upside of any trip abroad would be ruined by the anxiety I felt before flying/going away and during my holiday, knowing I had to fly home. The longer I did not fly, the bigger my fear grew. After I had my first child, the opportunity to go to Australia arose, and it was at this point that I recognized that this fear of flying was getting in the way of me **and** my family's life. I decided I needed to do something about it.

In life you might have situations that you avoid because of fear or anxiety. It might be that this has been triggered by difficult or traumatic experiences (where you felt fearful or out of control, like my plane journey) or it might have grown incrementally over time based on feelings and thoughts about hypothesized situations (e.g., being worried that you'll make a fool of yourself at a social event so you avoid going at all).

Most young people who are referred to me for support have got to the point where they are avoiding doing things that they are anxious or worried about. Typically, this has an impact on family life. The most common things children I work with avoid are going to school and taking part in social events. When our children stop doing these things, although temporarily it may offer them some relief from the worry, in the longer term, their anxiety about that thing grows and typically spreads to other situations. Below, you'll see the "Anxiety Trap" illustration, which highlights how this can become a vicious cycle.

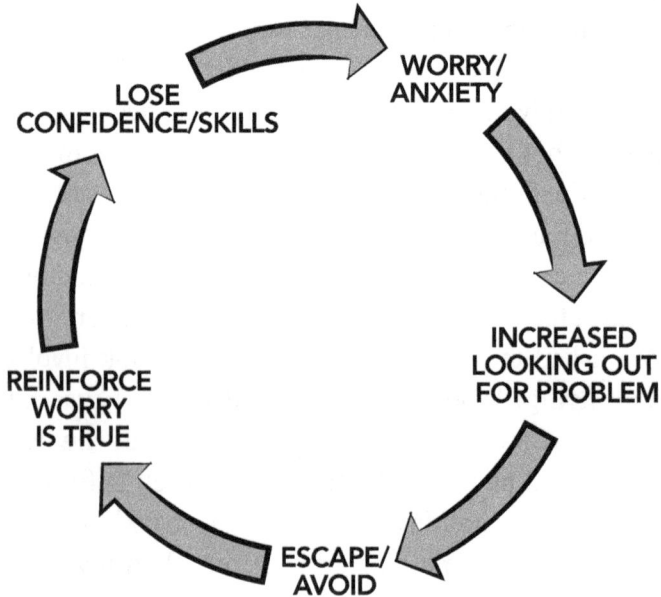

LOSE CONFIDENCE/SKILLS

WORRY/ ANXIETY

INCREASED LOOKING OUT FOR PROBLEM

REINFORCE WORRY IS TRUE

ESCAPE/ AVOID

Things we do that feed anxiety

In an attempt to reduce worry and/or take away the physical feelings of anxiety, there are a few behaviors we exhibit, such as:

* **avoidance**—not going into a feared situation (e.g., giving a friend's sleepover a miss);

* **escape**—stepping away from a feared situation or running away (e.g., leaving the classroom when starting to feel overwhelmed);

* **compensation**—doing more of something to reduce the possibility of a feared thing happening (e.g., washing hands more frequently to avoid germs);

* **safety behaviors**—engaging in habits or depending on things/people in order to feel safer or more prepared for a situation (e.g., relying on a mobile phone to look at rather than talking to others at a social event, staying close to a parent);

* **seeking reassurance**—asking others around us if things will be OK (e.g., asking a parent about upcoming events).

The above strategies can work quickly to reduce distress, which can be helpful for us in the moment, but they can pose a dilemma: how do we, as parents, respond when we see these behaviors in our children, particularly if they are presenting as very distressed? If we stop them from using the above strategies to cope, we may see an immediate increase in distress, which is very difficult for them and for us in the short term. At times, we might find ourselves encouraging some of these strategies to reduce distress and the possible fallout (e.g., not suggesting events to our children that might make them feel anxious, or reassuring them that they will be OK as we might be predicting that they will be worried). Try this exercise to work out what actions your child might be taking to manage the things they are worried or anxious about.

✏️

ACTIVITY BOX

Think of an activity or situation your child might be trying to avoid due to anxiety/worry. Use the worksheet in the resource pack to fill in the boxes below with your child. Ask your child, when they think about this situation, how they feel in their body (they can use the body picture on page 146 to point out how they feel), ask them to describe some of the thoughts they might have (e.g., I can't do it), and think with them about what they might do to cope with this activity/situation. I have filled in the table below with examples.

Body (how they feel)	Thoughts (what they think)	Behaviors (what they do)
Butterflies in tummy, headache	"I won't cope; something bad will happen."	Stay close to parent asking for reassurance. Refuse to attend school.

Facing our fears

The things we naturally do to reduce anxiety are both: (1) instinctual (if something is perceived as dangerous, the most effective way to stay safe is to get away from it); and (2) effective in the short term (they switch the stress response off), but as you can guess are less helpful in the longer term. As identified in chapter 7, modern-day life is relatively safe (unlike our Stone Age ancestors, we're not often exposed to physical threat), but we're constantly exposed to stressors that biologically feel like dangers to self. If our children use the strategies designed to protect them from being killed by saber-toothed tigers for their more typical daily stressors/worries (e.g., about academic and social performance), ironically this will likely decrease their safety in their world, rather than increase it. This is because, by avoiding or escaping the situations they are afraid of, they are not learning: (1) that the situation was safe enough and not as catastrophic as they feared (thereby not challenging their unhelpful thoughts); (2) that they *could* cope with the anxiety (thereby not learning to tolerate some physical anxiety); and (3) how to manage these feared situations well (thereby not learning the skills to support them to be successful in the things they care about).

Importantly, if these strategies are instinctual and effective in the short term, changing them to more helpful strategies in the long term requires plenty of conscious effort and motivation!

The families I meet with have usually arrived at a place where they've seen the cost of these strategies is impacting them in the long term. Their child will no longer go to school, is avoiding going out with friends or trying new things. Their world has gotten smaller and smaller. Typically, by this point, their child is not only anxious but also experiencing low mood. As a result, these children and their families are ready to seek another way to manage anxiety.

With my fear of flying, it was only when I recognized I wanted to go to Australia and provide rich opportunities for my child *more* than I wanted to listen to the worry, that I was willing to face my fear and do something to overcome it.

> **Reflection Box**
>
> Ask yourself: what incentivizes you to face your fears? (For example, feeling a sense of achievement, feeling valued by others, money, fear of the alternative.) Look back to the box on page 190 and the situation your child might be trying to avoid. What are the longer-term incentives for facing their fear(s) and going into the situation they are avoiding?

The power of doing what we're afraid of

Imagine being asked to prepare a presentation for work in front of a large audience on a topic that is not your speciality (75 percent of people have a fear of public speaking)! How would you feel? What would be going through your mind? What might you do to prepare for or avoid the presentation?

Imagine doing the presentation. How anxious would you feel about doing it, if you were to measure it on a scale of 1–10? Perhaps an 8 or 9? Let's say you complete the presentation and it isn't a disaster. How do you feel *now*? Envisage a supportive audience and your manager being pleased with the outcome. As a result, she asks you to repeat the presentation each morning for the following week. How anxious would you feel out of 10 on Tuesday about doing the presentation? Perhaps a 7? After another successful presentation experience, what about the next day? Maybe Wednesday, you might be around the 6 mark. By Friday, you would likely find your anxiety is at a 3 or 4 out of 10.

This is an example of **exposure** and **habituation**. When we're repeatedly exposed to something we're typically afraid of in a safe environment, it helps us overcome our fear.

In this scenario it works by:

* decreasing your fear reaction as you train your brain to reduce its stress response as well as unlearn negative associations (see the fact box below);

* challenging unrealistic or unhelpful thoughts/beliefs you might have about the feared situation (e.g., "I won't be able to speak to an audience"; "I'll forget everything"; "The audience will be bored or think I'm incompetent");

* building your skills to perform well in the feared situation (e.g., improvement in presentation skills).

-̣ᗧ̣- **Fact Box**

The single most effective way to overcome fear is by going into feared situations repeatedly and experiencing them as neutral or positive. This is because these experiences are literally changing the way our brain fires. As explained in chapter 7, the part of the brain linked to survival and emotional processing (the amygdala) is critical in sending distress signals to the brain when it's triggered by something it's afraid of. Research shows that providing repeated neutral or positive experiences of the thing that we're afraid of is effective in reducing the amount of distress signal the amygdala sends to the brain. For example, when people with phobic-level fear of spiders are shown repeated pictures of them, MRI scans show their amygdala reduces the amount of distress signal it produces—the brain essentially learns it no longer needs to be afraid of this thing as it has not hurt them.[49] Exposure to the previously feared thing in a safe environment enables the brain to build new meaning. It doesn't forget the old fear. We need the brain to be adaptive enough to recognize: I might not need to be scared of a house spider in my kitchen in the UK, but I might want to be cautious of a spider I come across in the Australian outback.

Graded exposure

In my work with young people, exposure plays a significant part of therapy. It's a vital element of the most effective therapy for treating anxiety disorders—Cognitive Behavioral Therapy (CBT)—with a recent research review finding that exposure was used in 91 percent of successful anxiety disorder treatments in children.[50] Young people I work with typically have fears that are too big to face in one go, so instead we work together to break down their feared situation into small steps, which means their exposure to the feared thing is gradual: this is called graded exposure. An example of how it's used with a young person is getting them to try doing a less-feared version of the thing they are afraid of and slowly working up to doing their most feared thing (e.g., looking at a picture of a spider, seeing a spider in a container, touching a spider).

As we raise our children, we will naturally be supporting them to grow and explore the world safely through graded exposure. Think about when you first taught your child to ride a bike. You might have started off by letting them play with a small balance bike (which allows them to walk with the bike between their legs and sit on the seat for brief periods of balance). Perhaps you bought your child their first bike in their favourite colour or one that features a much-loved character of theirs as well as stabilizers. You might have taught them in a garden or on a smooth pavement at a park, ensuring there is no danger of them losing control and being hurt by a car. If they fell and hurt themselves, you would pick them and their bike up and encourage them to get back on and try again, maybe with a little more help from you this time—running alongside them with your hand on the back of the seat to help them feel safe enough to enjoy the experience again. Gradually, you would build their skills and confidence up until they did not need stabilizers, could ride their bike on more adventurous and risky terrain, and, eventually, bike to wherever they need to go, such as school, independently (as my youngest now takes great pleasure in doing). The support and training you have instinctively provided your child with to get them to a place where they can independently and safely ride a bike is exposure and habituation. Helping your child experience as many times as they need to, feeling safe enough on their bike to be brave enough to tolerate the feeling of fear and uncertainty, while learning to develop the skills and confidence to embrace the exhilaration of movement on two wheels.

As parents, we're constantly juggling the balance between our instincts to protect and to enable our children to learn through their own experiences so they can develop independence and the ability to judge safe from unsafe. Often our own fears for our child, or our previous experiences, might impact our instinct to protect them, and we may unintentionally reinforce our child's perception of what's safe or unsafe. Imagine if you had never learned to ride a bike, or had experienced a bad bike crash as a child. Your approach to teaching your child to ride a bike would be influenced by these experiences.

The next section of this chapter will provide you with a practical tool to help you support your child to face their fears gradually: the brave behaviors ladder. As you use this tool with your child, think about the behaviors that would be most supportive in helping them to learn how to ride a bike. Apply these principles to supporting your children in doing the things they are afraid of. For example, exercising patience by not trying to do it for them, making it fun and collaborative, choosing the best time of day and right setting that is conducive to their learning, helping them get back on the bike when they experience setbacks, not leaving big gaps between rides, building time on their bike into their routine, tolerating your own anxiety and fears and not transferring them onto your child, not expecting your child to be able to ride a bike straight away and celebrating their small successes with pride and joy.

Acts of courage: A note on language

Anxiety and worry often create a sense of losing control. Many young people I work with believe that they are weak and have failed because they struggle with anxiety. I explain to young people and their parents that the way we use language is powerful. It can influence how children view themselves and what they consider themselves capable of. With a different choice of words we can go from perceiving ourselves as a victim of anxiety (e.g., "My anxiety stopped me going to school twice this week") to seeing ourselves as a survivor of anxiety (e.g., "I overcame my anxiety to get to school three days this week"). I remind young people to notice when they have anxious feelings in their body or worried thoughts, and tell them it's because they are about to do something brave, not necessarily because something bad is about to happen. Learning to live *with* anxiety, not *by* anxiety, can transform a child's view of themselves, and motivate them to stand up to the thing they are afraid of in pursuit of the person they want to be.

Most teenagers I work with long to feel more confident. They want to follow their dreams. In order to do great things, we all have to tolerate some anxiety. The better we can get at doing this, the stronger our confidence grows and we will start to notice the power of anxiety shrinking. Personally, the things that I've found most success in or that have brought me the most reward, I have felt scared about before doing them.

If you visit the stories of inspiring people throughout history, including our modern-day heroes, from Mother Teresa to Malala Yousafzai, you'll find that they all had to be brave, sit with uncertainty and live alongside any anxiety they might have felt (or feel) to do more of what counts for them.

Brave behaviors ladder

Take a look at the illustration on page 197. This is something I show young people, or ask that we draw together (see the resource pack for a worksheet you can use with your child). When I do this work with young people, we draw a ladder and work out what the goal of our work is and put this at the top.

We then work out the steps toward that goal. We start with things at the bottom of the ladder, which may raise some anxiety, but feel manageable, and gradually build up the tasks toward the most feared goal. The principle is that repetition of the feared situation will bring down our child's anxiety to a comfortable level. They can then move to the next rung of the ladder, and repeat this until their anxiety has reduced to an acceptable level. This experience will help give new meaning to the situation they previously feared, dispel beliefs about what might have happened and how well they would or wouldn't cope, and enable them to develop skills and confidence so that they can progress to doing other activities that might feel just outside of their reach.

To demonstrate this, I'll take you through how I used it with Noah from chapters 7 and 8. As you might recall, Noah was anxious about school and friendships. In chapter 7, he learned about how anxiety was triggering the stress response in his body and how to help his body settle down more quickly when starting to feel afraid, using slow breathing techniques, grounding exercises and physically exerting himself. In chapter 8, he learned that he tended to hypothesize the worst-case scenarios, which often triggered his stress response, and how to break free from the worry trap through problem-solving. We were now in a good place to think together about how Noah could do more of the things he wanted to do, despite feeling anxious about them, as he had learned coping strategies to help him face these fears.

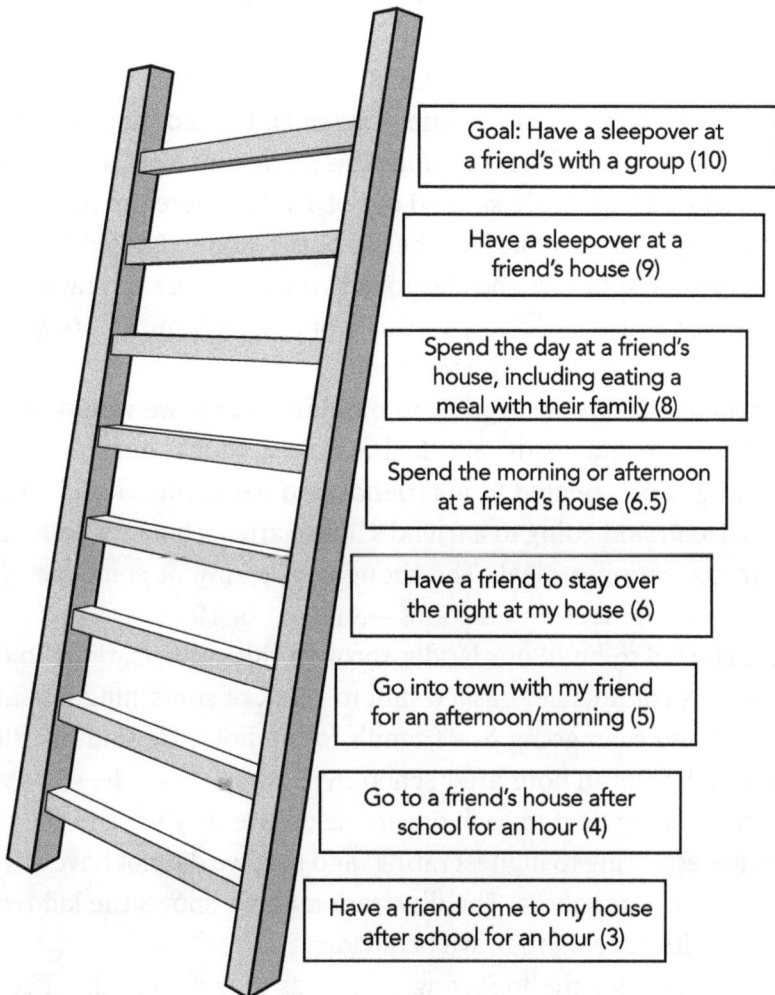

Goal: Have a sleepover at a friend's with a group (10)

Have a sleepover at a friend's house (9)

Spend the day at a friend's house, including eating a meal with their family (8)

Spend the morning or afternoon at a friend's house (6.5)

Have a friend to stay over the night at my house (6)

Go into town with my friend for an afternoon/morning (5)

Go to a friend's house after school for an hour (4)

Have a friend come to my house after school for an hour (3)

Noah identified that he had once stayed at a friend's house and had felt so homesick in the night that he had never been able to accept an invitation to stay at a friend's house since. This was causing wider problems—it meant he often made up elaborate stories when his friends were having sleepovers as to why he couldn't come and had missed a few events that his friends had invited him to (which involved both day activities and a sleepover). He would often worry about the next time his friends would ask him to stay over and how he could make up a believable excuse to not come. Later in the year, there was a residential trip at school and Noah did not have the confidence to sign up for it because he did not believe he could cope with being away from home overnight.

Noah and I started to build his ladder. His top goal was to be able to have a sleepover with a group of friends. I asked him to measure (on a scale from 1–10) how anxious this made him feel (see chapter 2 on scaling questions). He said 10 out of 10. We therefore agreed this was a good goal and wrote it at the top of the ladder. I asked him what the next feared thing around sleepovers would be. He said staying over at a friend's house on his own—this would be a 9 out of 10. We put this on the rung beneath the top one.

I explained if we were going to build up to this, we would need to try something that made him feel a little anxious, but felt doable, something which related to his friends and being round each other's houses. Noah said going to a friend's house after school for an hour or so, but not eating a meal. The thought of eating at someone else's house made him feel very anxious—an 8 out of 10.

We started to build our ladder through this conversation. To help improve his confidence, I asked him to think of something less anxiety-provoking than going to a friend's for an hour. He said his friend coming to his for an hour after school. We mapped out the steps with an anxiety rating next to each one to make sure they were in the right order, lowest rating to highest rating, and that we did not have any big jumps between numbers. The illustration above shows the ladder we came up with for Noah's brave behaviors.

Noah's task for the following week was to complete the first two rungs of his ladder. When I saw him in our next session, he had successfully completed these two things. I asked him how they had gone. He explained that both had gone well, though there were a few hiccups. They had been harder to organize than he'd thought, but his parents had been helpful, offering a lift to his friend. When I asked him to rate his anxiety for these two activities, rather than a 3 and a 4 out of 10 (as he had rated them before), they were now both a 2 out of 10.

We then looked at the next activity on the ladder: going into town with friends. We planned how he might do this and did some problem-solving together about possible barriers. I was able to remind Noah about continuing to use and practice his breathing techniques and grounding exercises, as well as writing out some helpful thoughts, to be able to reassure himself, such as:

* *My friends are kind. They like me.*
* *The more time I spend with my friends, the stronger our friend-ship and my confidence will grow and the easier it will get.*
* *I might feel scared, but that is just my brain trying to keep me safe.*
* *I'm safe.*

In this way, we were able to build up to Noah's goal of staying at a friend's house when invited to a party. Each rung of the ladder we had celebrated together in our sessions, but this final goal was such an achievement, he marked it with his family having a favorite takeaway so they could celebrate together just how brave he had been and how hard he had worked to achieve this goal. Later, Noah told me with great pride that he had signed up for the residential trip. He planned to have lots of overnight stays with friends to ensure he built up his confidence at sleeping away from home in preparation for the trip. Noah's gradual and consistent success fed his motivation to continue up the ladder and beyond.

If you do this exercise with your child, use the brave behavior activity sheet in the resource pack. If it's difficult for you to collabora-tively complete this task with your child, think about how you can integrate this graded approach to supporting your child over time to do more of the things they are anxious about. Again, using it for your-self and talking aloud throughout about how you're managing your own approach to anxiety-provoking situations is the most powerful way of teaching your child.

> ### ☁ Reflection Box
>
> Reflect on what activities or situations you might avoid due to anxiety or your fears and beliefs about what you're capable of. Build your own brave behaviors ladder. Approach the task recognizing the more visibly you can demonstrate how you tackle the things you're afraid of, the more your children will learn through your example.
>
> I often like to vocalize the process of making sense of my feelings with my children (e.g., saying aloud, "I'm really worried about a big presentation I have to do in a couple of weeks, so I need to make sure I practice it on my own, then in front of a friend, then in front of a work colleague. It won't take the anxiety away, but it will make it less scary. I know how good I'll feel after I've done this presentation, so it will be worth it").

Moving from reassurance to self-assurance

When I went on my first flight after five years of avoiding airplane travel, I spent a huge amount of energy seeking reassurance from oth-ers. I asked my then-husband, "It will be OK, won't it?" I sought advice from my friends before the build-up to the trip, saying, "Tell me it will be OK. You flew earlier this year and it was OK, wasn't it?" Every inter-action I had with airport staff or flight attendants, I was looking for some kind of guarantee that it would all be fine. I was hypervigilant in checking their body language, how relaxed they looked, to reassure me that this flight was going to be safe. I even told the flight attendant that I was terrified of flying and asked about possible turbulence. She went and spoke to the pilots and they invited me to visit them in the cockpit during the flight (this would never happen now due to increased security). The pilots were so relaxed I could hardly believe it. They told me how many flights they had done in their lives and that they had all been uneventful. I went back to my seat with a newfound confidence. At this point, I came to the realization that I cannot personally visit the cockpit of every future plane trip to ensure the competence of the pilots and the safety of the flight. However, despite this, a large part of me wanted to continue to depend on the confidence and reassurance of others rather than my own ability to calm myself.

As a parent, you might have experienced your child seeking frequent reassurance for things they are worried about. You will likely be on autopilot when it comes to comforting them, repeatedly replying, "Yes, it will be fine" and "No, you have nothing to worry about." The problem with reassurance is, like avoidance, it helps to provide some temporary relief from the distress your child is experiencing. However, in the long term, your child may become dependent on this reassurance to be able to go into situations they are uncertain about.

Naturally, we will often want to provide reassurance to those we have relationships with, but when you notice your child seeking reassurance repeatedly, and it seems to increasingly not be enough, a different approach might be required.

I often say to parents and young people that we all need to develop the skill of talking to ourselves in a supportive manner (self-compassion). This can be a really difficult habit to get into. Research shows that writing down our thoughts and feelings on a daily basis can help improve our wellbeing, increase resilience, and decrease stress[51] (see gratitude activities on page 184). Getting into the habit, or encouraging your child to get into the habit of journaling, can support the development of self-compassion, as well as provide an opportunity to process and express difficult feelings.

When your child is seeking reassurance, you can try the following steps to help them develop the skill of self-assurance. If your child practices this repeatedly, it can grow to become their own internal voice that they can listen to when they feel uncertain or anxious. It's this voice that will help guide them forward and encourage the self-belief or confidence to do the thing they are anxious about.

Top tips for moving your child from reassurance to self-assurance

- ► Listen to your child's worries in an open way.

- ► Make time for this—picking the moment (see page 111 for top tips on this).

- ► Encourage them to answer their own questions.

- ► Ask them what they think the likelihood is of something bad happening.

- ► Encourage them to come up with ideas, including things that have worked before, for solving their worries and reassuring themselves.

- ► Support them to break things down into achievable tasks, least feared first.

Building resilience

As we come to the end of part 3, let's revisit what we've learned about anxiety when it comes to stopping it from controlling your child's life. I want to reflect on something of relevance from part 2, where we looked at difficult feelings. When our children are in distress, firstly, we need to sit alongside them and see and acknowledge their distress without trying to move them on too quickly from this. If your child feels seen and understood, this will immediately lead to a de-escalation of their physical response. They will then be in a better place to take on any thinking or talking or making sense of what comes now and what comes next (connection before correction).

As explored in chapter 6, so often we do not want our children to experience difficult emotions; we want to take these feelings or fears away and/or solve the problem. But learning to go through this emotion and understanding it's safe to do so can help a young person develop resilience and a sense that when hard things happen, they have the skills to deal with them.

As parents, we don't have to pretend we know everything, or that we have control over everything. The key is to show up and see our children fully, while exploring the idea of asking for and accepting help from others as a positive life skill. Not a failure.

Through doing the activities that I have shared here with many young people, I've often discovered that their anxiety or strong feelings reflect a *skill* deficit, rather than a *will* deficit. That is, they are struggling in a particular area because they need support to develop skills in that area. Their reluctance to do the tasks is because of this skill deficit rather than them not wanting to do the task. This may be particularly relevant for children with neurodevelopmental diversity or additional needs.

Our children building resilience relies on them having repeated experiences of success when doing things that feel difficult. We build resilience through experience, one success at a time. The important thing to hold in mind is that we're supporting our children to do things that are within their reach. Think about teaching your child to swim. You remove their buoyancy aids or increase the depth of the pool once you can see that they've learned how to swim unaided. If we recognize our child has difficulties with controlling their breathing in the water or coordination, we don't just take the buoyancy aids away when it suits us. Instead, we provide our child with additional practice and encouragement to help them build their confidence and skills, despite their vulnerability. The same is true more generally. Think about your child's strengths and other areas where they might struggle. Find ways to use their strengths to their advantage (stubbornness is a great strength which can be used positively in the pursuit of not giving up doing the things that count). Let's not unintentionally set our kids up to fail. If our children need help developing social skills in order to have a better chance of success on their brave behavior ladder for spending more time with friends, explore how you or others can support your child develop these social skills. If your child struggles with organization, writing, or reading and this difficulty is affecting their experience of school, explore what opportunities they have to do more of these things within their zone of achievement, to help them build these skills and have more opportunities for success in these areas. Just as we wouldn't leave the buoyancy aids on our child even when they've learned to swim independently, we must ensure we don't unintentionally hold our children back with our own fears and anxieties about them doing more of the things they find hard.

SUMMARY

→ When we feel afraid or worried about something, instinct tells us to avoid that thing or try to escape it.

→ Avoiding things that make us distressed offers short-term relief, but in the long term increases anxiety.

→ When our children avoid things that are not going to hurt them (e.g., like going to school), they are not learning:

- that the situation was not as catastrophic as they feared;
- that they could cope with the anxiety;
- the skills to cope with these feared situations.

→ Helping our children to recognize that often, when we notice an anxious feeling in our bodies, it's because we're about to do something brave, can reframe their view of themselves.

→ Supporting our children in doing things that are important to their development and growth, but that they are anxious about, through breaking these things down into manageable steps is a helpful way to break the cycle of avoidance.

→ As parents, we can provide our child with the skills to self-assure rather than rely on us for reassurance in the way we respond to our child's fears.

→ Making sure we support our children in developing the necessary skills to meet these challenges will help them experience success in taking on challenging tasks, especially if a child has neurodevelopmental diversity (e.g., Autism Spectrum Condition, ADHD) or has experienced trauma.

→ If our children learn to do the things they are anxious about, their experience of success will build confidence and resilience to face the challenges of life.

PART 4
Low Mood

How to get your child back

Chapter 10

Low-mood traps

"I just don't want my parents to know how bad I'm feeling. It will make things worse."

Time and time again I hear these words from the young people who come to my office, confused and lonely: they are not coping. Their parents are often equally confused and worried about their child, who no longer seems as interested in life and is harder to reach. "I just wish he would tell me what's going on, then we can try to help," they say. They look to me to solve the mystery, sometimes hoping I can fix the problem, but other times just wanting to be given reassurance and guidance on how to support their child.

In part 4, we'll be exploring the queries you might have as a parent about low mood or depression. This section of the book provides practical approaches to help you support your child in boosting their mood and motivation for life; whether they are experiencing a one-off bad day or struggling with more persistent low mood. This chapter explains low mood, what it might look like in your child and gives an insight into why the adolescent brain is particularly susceptible to mood fluctuations, as well as the red flags for depression.

Why low mood?

Throughout their youth everyone will at one point or another experience low mood, sadness, irritability, not wanting to be with others and loss of interest in things they enjoy. Usually, such feelings will be linked to the trials and tribulations of life. They will come and go, like waves; perhaps a few minutes or hours of the day, perhaps the odd day in a week. In these moments, as a parent, you might feel frustrated, as you'll find your child/adolescent hard to communicate with and lacking in energy and enthusiasm. You might also worry about whether the way your child is feeling is normal or perhaps a sign of deeper difficulties with their wellbeing.

Feeling low or sad is a natural—and necessary—part of life. Sadness is an emotion that tells us something in our life is not right. Like all emotions, sadness has a purpose. It's a response to situations where we might experience loss (e.g., loss of a relationship, financial security or social status). How it affects us physically is designed to help us initially conserve energy (to prevent more loss and provide space for healing) and then motivate us to recover the lost thing (seek out the other person, increase income, repair the relationship). Sadness is an emotion felt and displayed in the body (e.g., downcast face, tears, body posture). This means it's recognized by others and can be a useful signal for help, to either retrieve what's lost, or receive comfort to relieve some of the pain of the loss (as shown in the diagram, below).

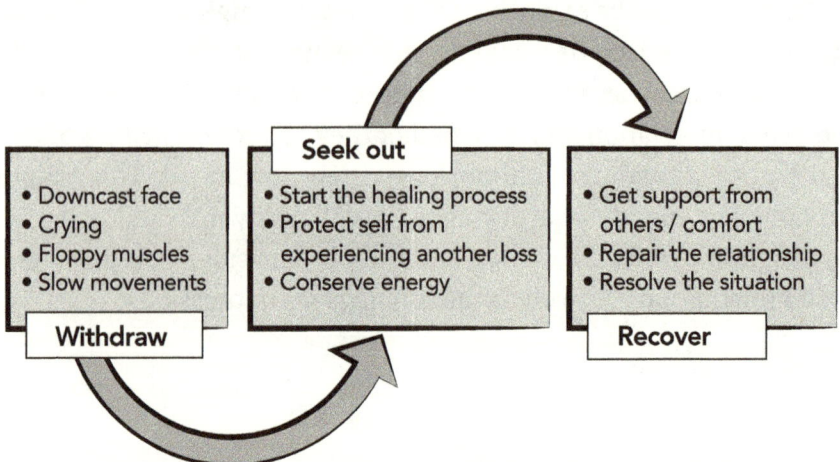

Withdraw
- Downcast face
- Crying
- Floppy muscles
- Slow movements

Seek out
- Start the healing process
- Protect self from experiencing another loss
- Conserve energy

Recover
- Get support from others / comfort
- Repair the relationship
- Resolve the situation

> **☁ Reflection Box**
>
> Think of something that has made you feel sad.
>
> Was it related to a loss or possible loss in your life?
>
> How did it make your body feel?
>
> What type of thoughts did you have?
>
> What did you initially do when you felt sad?
>
> What helped relieve the sadness?

Low mood and sadness can be brought on by **external stressors** in our lives (the things that happen to us), and **internal stressors** (our thoughts; questions about our identity, worth, and purpose). Typically, these stressors are likely to put in jeopardy the important areas below:

* **relationships** (connections with others, loving and being loved, friendship, sense of belonging);

* **staying safe** (security, safe place to live, nourishment, being warm and comfortable, health, parental mental health, not being hurt physically or emotionally);

* **doing meaningful activities** (learning, having a sense of purpose, achievement, making a difference, caring for others);

* **feeling pleasure and enjoyment.**

For some young people, low mood may come out of nowhere, but for most, there will be an event in their life that can be linked to a change in their mood. Look at the table below. These are reasons parents felt concerned about their child's low mood. Does your child's low mood make sense in the context of these situations?

ACTIVITY BOX

Note from the table below the situations you recognize might be having an impact on your child's mood. Consider which of the seven Wellbeing Abacus areas (page 37) these situations jeopardize. If you've completed chapter 6's activity on exploring your child's values (page 124), consider whether the situations you have selected link to your child's values/what's important to them, as seen in the example below.

Feeling different	Gender identity	Sexuality	Loneliness	Lack of sleep
Bereavement	School pressures	Cyber-bullying	Verbal abuse	Failure
Family health	Transitions/change	Body image	Social exclusion	Hormones
Boredom	Parental conflict	Romantic issues	No job	Isolation
Loss	Bullying	Existential crisis	Money worries	Learning difficulties
Wellbeing Abacus areas affected?		e.g., connect with others, sleep		
What's important to my child?		e.g., loyalty, belonging, feeling loved		

What does low mood look like in my child?

There are a number of things that you might notice happen to your child's mood, thinking and activity levels when they are feeling low. Look at the ones that you might notice in your child in the table below.

Mood	Thinking	Activity
• Sadness • Increased irritability • Things don't feel as much fun anymore • Loss of interest in activities	• Difficulty making decisions • Poor concentration • Self-critical focus • Feeling worthless • Thoughts of death	• No energy • Increased tiredness • Restless • Slowed down • Appetite changes • Sleep changes • Pain

When our mood, thinking and activity levels are affected in the way described in the table for longer periods of time, we can become trapped in the "conserving energy" phase of sadness, which can prevent us from having enough energy or motivation to move to the phase where we might take action to resolve the difficulty. If we get trapped in this phase, the things we do when we feel low can add to feeling this way. For example:

* If we don't find things as much fun anymore and we have less energy, we might stop doing the things that we enjoy or are important to us.

* If others irritate us more and we feel worthless, we might withdraw from others and thus reduce our opportunity for support and social connection.

* If we get stuck in negative thoughts or become more focused on what's not going well for us, this can reinforce a sense of hopelessness and helplessness.

In trying to protect us from emotional pain or further losses, low mood can stop us doing what we need to do to feel better.

☁ Reflection Box

Remember a time when your child felt sad in the days following losing something important in their life (e.g., a loved one dying—this could be a person or a pet; not seeing someone they care about—a parent, a friend). Remember how your child responded. They might have spent more time on their own or perhaps been clingier. They could have lost interest in food or wanted to eat for comfort. Maybe they experienced difficulty getting to sleep, or waking up with bad dreams, or had less energy and wanted to sleep more. You may have found they weren't interested in the things they usually enjoy, perhaps meeting up with others or even watching their favorite TV show. They may have appeared to be preoccupied with a heaviness that seemed to drag them down. As a parent, you would see all these things and understand this was their response to the sadness and distress they were feeling because of their loss. Seeing them like this would have prompted you to be more available to them, offering them warmth and care and encouraging them to do some things you know would cheer them up. You might have offered space to talk about the loss and helped them make sense of what it means to them. Their physical manifestation of sadness would prompt you to take action to support them through these tricky hours and days as they came to terms with the loss. The things you do and how they respond would help them recover from the loss and get back to engaging with and enjoying life. However, if they were unresponsive to your attempts, and persisted with all these things (not doing things they enjoy, staying on their own, suffering disturbed patterns of eating and sleeping), it would move from their sadness driving their disengagement with their life, to their disengagement from life driving the sadness—thus creating the low-mood trap.

Do I need to worry about my child?

Many families I meet have noticed their child is stuck in a low mood that won't go away. It prevents them doing the things they need to do in their life (e.g., completing schoolwork, spending time with others).

Often these parents are scared as they don't understand what's going on inside their child and they don't know what to do to help. It's at this point that the child and/or parent will ask me if I think they are depressed or just low.

Clinical depression, as defined by the diagnostic manuals produced by the WHO (World Health Organization) and APA (American Psychiatric Association), is different from normal sadness or low mood in the below three ways:

1. *Number of signs and symptoms*
   Depression would require that a young person was experiencing five of the signs/symptoms listed in the mood-thinking-activity table (page 211), with at least one being sadness, irritability, or loss of interest in activities.

2. *Duration*
   Depression is a continuous state and therefore these five signs/symptoms would need to be experienced nearly every day for most of the day, for at least two weeks.

3. *Impact*
   Depression has a big impact on life. Young people with depression would be struggling to engage with daily activities of life. This would negatively impact school (or work) and relationships.

Often the challenge for a parent is filling in the gaps, as children or adolescents are not likely to describe everything they are feeling. Many young people have mastered the art of hiding how difficult things are for them internally; they might be trying to protect the adults around them from worry, or fear that revealing their struggles will not get the response they need from others. This is where being curious about changes in your child's behavior can be important clues as to what could be going on for them and whether they need more support (e.g., unexpectedly withdrawing from their friends or family members, stopping doing things they previously enjoyed, changes in sleep or eating patterns, changes in energy levels). A change in one of these areas wouldn't be as concerning as a number of these changes happening at the same time, particularly if you can see it's having a negative impact on your child's ability to engage with their life.

Depression can be a difficult feeling for young people to describe, often because it's an absence of expected feelings rather than a great sense of sadness. For some, their experiences will create emotions that are so painful that repressing, or pushing them deeper inside, becomes the only way to survive the pain. This lack of opportunity to express, make sense of these feelings and give meaning to the difficult experience that created the feelings, leads to a cutting-off not only of the painful emotions, but all emotions—leaving an emptiness or numbness.

Chronic stress can play a role, with a body–mind shutdown becoming a protective mechanism from continued and ongoing stress. On page 102, in the window of tolerance, you can see how a prolonged period of being hyperaroused can lead to exhaustion of the nervous system. In order to defend itself, it moves to the protective state of hypoarousal; essentially shut down.

Losing access to the range of emotions that support our wellbeing and sense of being alive naturally leads to feelings of disconnection and helplessness, where a young person may feel they are no longer able to effect change in their life. From this can arise a sense of hopelessness about the future. This internal pain and difficulty in expressing distress can lead to self-harm and suicidal thoughts, which are explored in more detail in chapter 12.

It's painful imagining how hard your child might be finding life if they get to this place of depression. It might hurt even more if you recognize some of these ways of coping with difficult feelings are ways you've survived loss in your own life.

In part 2, we explored the power of connection and how making sense of difficult experiences and feelings can help a young person recover from difficult events. This guidance is important as it explains how giving young people the opportunity to feel heard and valued and that their feelings matter can itself be transformational. One young person said to me: "You may never know the impact of a conversation on someone else. I'm grateful to a person I only met once for being able to talk to them. It saved my life, really."

The remainder of this part of the book complements the advice in part 2. It includes information and tools that are proven to help low mood or depression in both young people and adults, which, applied with the principles of part 2, creates a strong foundation for supporting your child more practically.

Clinical Depression Q&A

Q: How many people struggle with depression?

A: Across the world 280 million people suffer from depression. Globally, it's a leading cause of disability.[52] Adolescents are the most likely to have experienced one episode of major depressive disorder (14 percent), compared to children (1 percent) and adults (7.1 percent).

Q: If either of my child's parents has struggled with depression, will that mean my child also will?

A: The strongest risk factors for depression in adolescence are a family history of depression and experiencing psychosocial stress. An adolescent with a parent with depression is three to four times more likely to experience depression. Growing up in a warm and loving environment and reducing a child's exposure to chronic stress helps reduce the risk of depression.

Q: *What might put my young person more at risk for developing depression?*

A: *The causes of depression are still not well understood. But there are both biological and social influences. Some things that have been shown to increase the risk of depression include: parent having/had depression; acute stressful events like bereavement; chronic adversity like bullying or neglect; and being female.*

Q: *What protects young people from depression?*

A: *The things that help protect against depression include general intellectual ability, good emotional regulation, healthy ways of coping with stress, positive thinking styles, and good-quality relationships with others. See the Wellbeing Abacus for more.*

Q: *If my adolescent has depression, will it mean they will have it forever? Will they be more prone to it in the future?*

A: *Your adolescent will not have depression forever, but they are more likely to have another episode of depression in the future than an adolescent who has not suffered with depression.*

Q: *Is it true that depression is because of a chemical imbalance in the brain?*

A: *The idea that depression is linked to lower serotonin levels in the brain has been around for decades. However, the most recent research suggests that that this is not the case. Often the belief that depression is the result of a chemical imbalance encourages people to consider medication as the only way to treat depression and makes them less likely to believe that they can do things to improve their mood.[53] It's becoming more widely accepted that the body–mind link is very complex, with physiology and environment impacting one another. This means that abnormalities in how neurotransmitters might work are not simply a product of our biology, but also how our experiences influence our biology. This understanding can help us move away from a deficit model, "What's wrong with me?" to "What's happened to me? What's my story? What's my family story? And, most importantly, what matters to me?"[54]*

Q: Is my adolescent more likely to end their life if they have a diagnosis of depression?

A: Adolescents with a diagnosis of depression are at increased risk of attempting and completing suicide. They are also at increased risk of self-harm and substance misuse (using drugs or alcohol).

Q: Do prescribed drugs help depression in young people?

A: Studies have shown that antidepressants can be effective in reducing symptoms of depression in adolescents. However, the effectiveness may vary among individuals and may not work for everyone. There are potential risks associated with antidepressants, including the risk of side effects and suicidal thoughts. Ideally, a young person diagnosed with moderate to severe depression would need an assessment by a child and adolescent psychiatrist to be considered for an antidepressant drug and would require monitoring by their healthcare team. It is recommended a child or adolescent should have a talking therapy (like Cognitive Behavioral Therapy) even if they were prescribed an antidepressant medication.[55]

If you're worried about your child and you feel they need access to more support, head to page 307 for signposting.

What can we do to help?

Prevention

As discussed in chapters 7 and 8, our modern environment is often mismatched with how our minds and bodies evolved to live in the Stone Age. Rather than spending our time in small communities prioritizing hunter-gathering activities, which would have involved physical tasks and spending most of our time outdoors, today our children are growing up in a world of multiple pressures. With plentiful access to a range of food and substances that are not always good for them and much bigger and more complex communities (family, school, work, social media), it can be overwhelming for us all. As outlined in chapter 3, access to some of the positive parts of progress (e.g., technology) can become stressors in themselves.

Dr. Steve Ilardi, an American clinical psychologist, has identified six areas (diet, exercise, meaningful activity, sunlight exposure, social connection, sleep) that protect against low mood.[56] These six areas are consistent with the seven areas covered in chapter 2's Wellbeing Abacus. In the table below, consider one small change you could make to support your child or yourself to promote an anti-low-mood lifestyle in your family.

Anti-low-mood lifestyle with the Wellbeing Abacus

Connect with others: Critical for wellbeing. Peer relationships and social status are particularly important for adolescents.

Physical activity: More movement and physical activity can reduce the impact of stress, and improve mood and physical health.

Sleep: Low mood impacts sleep quality and in turn contributes to low mood. Supporting good sleep is protective for both mental and physical health. It can be a particular challenge for adolescents—how you can help is covered below.

Nutrition: Increased omega-3 fatty acid foods/supplements with their anti-inflammatory properties can reduce the impact of stress on the nervous system. Not getting enough sunshine can contribute to low mood. Brain serotonin is at its lowest in the winter and highest in the summer. Getting outside, a light box, and vitamin D all help.

Take notice: Opportunities to engage in "flow" activities (see page 73).

Top Tips: Sleep

Bedroom:

► Reduce the light at night; increase the light in the morning.

► Temperature—people sleep better in a cool environment, so check that your child's room is not too hot.

Food and drink:

► Avoid caffeine in food and drinks in the afternoon and evening.

► Hunger—avoid going to bed hungry.

Routines:

► Making routines that help our bodies know they need to prepare for sleep is helpful. Create a "wind-down" hour or two before bed—this can help the body relax and feel sleepy. Winding down can involve activities which are soothing and not too stimulating, such as calm talking to others, listening to relaxing sounds, or having a warm shower/bath (which lowers your body's core temperature, aiding sleep). Mindfulness and sleep meditations have become increasingly popular and exercises can be freely accessed through apps. Using the same sound/music every night and/or a special scent (e.g., lavender) can help the brain associate these sensory cues with sleep.

► Use a flexible routine—this means aiming to go to bed and waking up at a similar time each day. Try to avoid lie-ins that are more than two hours later than when normally needing to wake up.

► If your child lies in bed for long periods without falling asleep you may need to make their bedtime later, and only go to bed at the point they need to go to sleep. For example, for nine hours' sleep if they need to wake up at 7 a.m., it may be that they shouldn't go to bed until 10 p.m. This will protect them from lying in bed for long periods not sleeping, where they learn to associate being in bed with not sleeping and/or feeling stressed about sleep.

► Bedrooms are often used for a range of activities. Try to ensure children use their bed for sleep and not other activities. The body–mind needs to associate the bed with sleep (not watching TV or playing games or lying awake feeling anxious). Try to pack things out of sight at sleep time that might be a distraction or trigger worries about the next day.

► With older children, avoid daytime napping.

Worry:

► Worry about not having a good night's sleep can increase stress and disrupt sleep. Use the tips in part 3 of the book to help encourage the relaxation response (e.g., practice deep breathing at night).

► Reduce the thoughts or situations that increase the stress response in the evening (e.g., keep conflict low, allow time earlier in the day to talk about [or write down] worries or struggles using the tools in chapter 8).

Changing a sleep pattern:

► Gradually shift the sleep cycle if you want to help your child sleep earlier so they can wake up earlier. Changes of fifteen to thirty minutes every few days can help gradually shift the sleeping pattern.

► Resist the urge to force sleep. When we wake up in the night, it's very frustrating and it can be natural to tell ourselves or our children to just try to go back to sleep. However, if we're alert and not sleepy then this will likely only cause more frustration. Although it feels counterintuitive, it can be more helpful to get out of bed and do something which is not too stimulating and does not involve bright lights, until you start to feel sleepy again.

Adolescence and low mood

The period of adolescence holds the greatest risk for low mood to develop, with adolescents experiencing the highest rates of depression across all age groups. As covered in detail in chapter 14, adolescence is a time of great physical change, both in terms of puberty (hormonal changes) and brain restructuring. It also is a time of increased expectations, with an emphasis on the growth of independence and a change in social priorities (moving toward friends and romantic relationships and away from family). These biological and social changes influence our adolescents' motivations as well as how they experience their world and its stressors, increasing their vulnerability to mental health difficulties.

As outlined in chapter 14, adolescent brains go through a significant restructure. These changes influence the way the upstairs and downstairs brain communicate with each other. Adolescence is therefore a time when young people will experience more extreme emotions, be inclined to take more risks and have a need to take part in exciting activities. They will also be more concerned about their social world compared to adults.

All these brain changes provide opportunities for our teenagers, but also mean they can be especially sensitive to what's happening in their world. Importantly, this combination of ripeness for learning and sensitivity to their world means that their brains are very responsive to the support we can provide as adults.

Mood and the three Rs

Changes in the adolescent brain impact mood through the three Rs: rewards, relationships and rumination, as explained in more detail here.

Rewards: Did you notice that as your child became a teenager the things they seemed to enjoy changed? Do they complain of being bored when not doing their preferred activities? Brain science can help explain this. We know reward and activity brain circuits change during adolescence. This is a necessary part of development to motivate adolescents to try new things so they become more independent from their families. To assist them in this, the feel-good neurochemical dopamine has a different impact on the brain during adolescent years.

Although the neuroscience in this area is still evolving, some research suggests that the changing influence of dopamine on the adolescent brain can affect how stimulating some activities are.[57] Essentially, this suggests that adolescents might need more of the right stimulation (rewards) to feel good, meaning they are especially dependent on new, positive experiences to thrill and excite them. Therefore, what our adolescents spend their time doing—or not doing—can have a big impact on their mood, as well as their brain development.

Relationships: Do you notice that your teenager is preoccupied with how others perceive them or what's happening in their social group? Does being "left out" or friendship difficulties have a disproportionately negative impact on their mood and stress levels? Again, these changes you might notice are influenced by what's happening in the brain. Adolescent brains are wired to be particularly sensitive to social rewards and negative social feedback. This sensitivity is nature's way of keeping them safe from others who might be a threat to them and encourages prosocial behavior (as they are no longer relying on their parents so much to do this for them). This means adolescents are likely to have a preoccupation with fitting in and a fear of exclusion from their peer group. As the adolescent brain is more affected by both negative (e.g., parental conflict, bullying) and positive interpersonal experiences (e.g., warm caregivers, being part of a friendship group), their social world has a huge impact on their mood.

Rumination: Do you notice your adolescent might focus on negative details and overly dwell on these? Again, brain science can help us understand this. As explored in chapter 8, the negative-bias thinking habits we get stuck in can greatly influence our mood. During adolescence the brain creates stronger neural networks for the things it does more. It therefore gets better at doing these things. The habits we form in adolescence are likely to be habits we continue into adulthood. For young people who get into the habit of ruminating (dwelling on negative thoughts), their neural connections increase to support this habit. The habit of rumination is linked to low mood and depression in adolescents and adults.[58] Research shows that supporting reduction of rumination: (1) changes neural connectivity (breaks the habit); (2) protects against (prevents) low mood and depression; and (3) if a young person has depression, leads to improvement.

Low mood	Additional adolescent brain challenges	Ways to help
Less reward out of life	Need more thrills to experience reward, more sensitive to social rewards	Structure, meaningful activity planning (chapter 11)
Relationship difficulties/ withdrawal	Peer relationships critical, adult input less valued, more sensitive to negative social cues, feels emotions more intensely, may maintain a persona of doing well	Supporting connection and communication skills (part 2, chapters 11 and 13)
Increased rumination	Negativity bias, hypersensitive to negative social feedback, social narrative around "perfection'	Unhooking from unhelpful thoughts (chapters 8 and 11)

Puberty: The added challenge of being female

Across the life span, post-pubertal women experience higher levels of anxiety and depressive disorders compared to post-pubertal boys and men. If you have a daughter who has gone through puberty (typically aged 12+), she's three times more likely to experience depression than a brother of the same age. Although this is a complex area with many unanswered questions, research suggests hormones play a role in this difference. During puberty, girls' bodies produce more estrogen (the main female sex hormone needed for puberty, the menstrual cycle and pregnancy) and boys produce more testosterone (the main male sex hormone needed for the development of the testes and prostate, as well as increased muscle and bone mass, and growth of body hair). These hormones play an important role, both in preparing the body for reproduction and determining how the body (central nervous system) responds to stress.

Some studies have found that fluctuations in estrogen can increase the stress response's (page 144) sensitivity to stress, perhaps increasing adolescent girls'/women's risk of mood disorders. In contrast, testosterone production can protect the body from stress, perhaps buffering adolescent boys/men from the risk of mood disorders. It is important to be aware that chronic stress can impact the production of oestrogen, testosterone, and other important hormones.

It's essential for girls and women to understand how hormonal cycles may influence their mental health, so they can make sense of some of the unique challenges they face depending on their menstrual cycle and the time of life when hormonal fluctuations tend to be bigger (e.g., adolescence, the perinatal and perimenopausal period). A conversation with your family doctor if you are worried about this can be invaluable.

- -

CASE STUDY

Charlie's Story (Part 1): The low-mood trap

In this story, we will follow Charlie, an adolescent stuck in the low-mood trap.

Charlie is a fourteen-year-old boy in Year Ten. He has started to notice that he's generally feeling low, and it's beginning to impact school life. He describes feeling irritated by everything, even his friends, having a lack of energy in the day and trouble sleeping at night, as well as not enjoying the things that he used to, like gaming and meeting up with friends.

He has a sense of not being good enough and wants to spend more time on his own, as everything feels too difficult. At home his parents have noticed he is mostly in his room and when he isn't he gets upset with others quickly. He isn't participating in family activities he used to enjoy, such as going out for lunch. There are more arguments at home because Charlie wants to be left alone and his parents (who are very supportive and worried about him) keep asking him what's wrong and getting upset when he says "nothing; leave me alone."

Charlie felt this had all come from nowhere, but we were able to do a timeline and work out that this feeling hadn't come out of the blue. It started with Charlie's grandmother dying, which had made him feel sad. The sadness didn't go away like he hoped and the things Charlie stopped doing temporarily (going to the gym regularly, meeting up with friends), he didn't start again. He noticed he felt bored by everything, and would choose to be on his own because he found himself paying so much attention to any signs that his friends did not like him, which was too stressful to bear. With less to do, he tended to use his time getting caught up with thinking about his gender identity and how he felt different to others, which in turn made him feel worse.

- -

Getting out of the low-mood trap

Like many young people and adults I meet, Charlie is stuck in the low-mood trap. As a parent, it can feel very difficult to know how to facilitate your child to get out of this, especially as low mood can make it harder to connect.

Using the tools in part 2 to connect and provide a safe space to express, validate, and make sense of feelings is a critical part of the process of understanding and supporting a young person. Alongside this, there are practical ways that Charlie and others can get out of the low-mood trap. These ways involve the 3 Rs:

* **Rewards**: Increase opportunity for doing healthy activities that feel good.

* **Relationships**: Increase and improve social connection with others.

* **Rumination**: Reduce the habit of rumination and getting stuck in negative thinking.

These approaches support the body–mind balance, as well as help our children to understand how low mood can impact their Wellbeing Abacus. They provide the tools for insight and action, expression and healing. In chapter 11, we will explore how you can practically support your child in these three areas.

SUMMARY

→ Sadness and low mood are normal human reactions to stressors and events in our lives.

→ Sadness is an important emotion to help in situations of loss. It works initially to help us conserve energy and then seek out what we have lost.

→ The things we do when we experience sadness or low mood can unintentionally feed the low mood and not help us resolve the issue or heal from the event that may have caused emotional pain.

→ Depression is different to low mood in the number of activities it disrupts, its duration (more than two weeks), persistence (across multiple areas of life most days, every day) and how it affects our ability to do daily activities.

→ Supporting prevention of low mood through an anti-low-mood lifestyle can help build in good habits to promote activities that support the mind–body balance.

→ Adolescents are particularly prone to difficulties with low mood due to the physical and social changes they experience.

→ Low mood and depression can be helped with support in three areas: increasing rewards through activity, improving relationships and social connection and reducing the habit of rumination (going over negative thoughts over and over).

Chapter 11
Doing what counts

When my youngest son, at nine years old, said, "I wish I was dead," my heart sank. I had noticed he had not been his usual self for a few weeks. He seemed sad and withdrawn. It had started with him complaining about school. Not his friends, which he had lots of, but the lessons. He described what sounded like boredom to me, feeling frustrated stuck in one room all day with a teacher he did not gel with. What began as him not wanting to go to school had crept into not wanting to go to football (something he loved). Previously a very active child, he seemed to have no energy or enthusiasm for anything. He just wanted to be in his room, watching his favorite shows repeatedly. When he was with the rest of the family he would fly off the handle at the smallest thing, ending up in a fit of rage or tearful. Seeing my son become a shadow of himself, constantly swinging between sadness and rage, was heartbreaking. The main problem seemed to be school, but I knew I couldn't just magic him to a different school. As a parent, I wanted to know what I needed to do to help him get back to the energetic, fun-loving boy I knew.

During the first lockdown, I had seen a similar pattern of withdrawal from life in my two eldest children. Once the novelty of not having to go to school wore off, the lack of structure and meaningful activity led to my teenagers being lost in the loneliness of the day. With no school to get up for, they were going to bed later and waking up later. With no one to see, there was little point getting dressed. My eldest son relied on connecting with his friends through gaming and the joy of cooking, but this wasn't enough for his fifteen-year-old brain to feel fulfilled. My daughter depended on Netflix box sets and Snapchat with her friends, but with nothing to look forward to, I felt the general apathy and sense of sadness that life—for them and for everyone else—was not what it had been. When school opened up for children of key workers, they begrudgingly attended. The result was that I saw an immediate improvement in their sleep patterns, energy levels and engagement with learning and home life. This proved to me that how we spend our time impacts our mood and activity levels. This is something I knew as a psychologist, but had not previously experienced so starkly with my own children.

During the COVID-19 pandemic, many people experienced a negative shift in their wellbeing and will have noticed increased periods of low mood. This is reflected in a 77 percent increase in referrals to mental health services for young people compared to before the pandemic.[59] This was particularly true for teenagers and makes sense when we consider the impact of the loss of structure, meaningful activities, sense of freedom, autonomy, and social contact. For many, such losses will have led to increased feelings of loneliness and social isolation and a decreased sense of belonging and purpose. These losses would have led to fewer opportunities for reward and more opportunities to focus on the negative, two areas we will explore in this chapter.

The power of rewards

Rewards are incredibly powerful. The majority of things that we do, particularly if they are unpleasant or difficult, we do because we know that we will receive something in recognition of our work, efforts, or achievements. Rewards not only help us work toward a goal and get through difficult things; they also help us manage our mood.

Typically, we need rewards to counterbalance some of the challenges we face in life. When I'm having a difficult day, I often motivate myself to get through it with ideas of treats to help me recover or provide me with comfort. For me this could be chocolate, a glass of wine, a bath or watching a film. Simply believing that the difficulty I'm facing will in itself teach me something new or result in a better outcome can spur me on and improve the amount of effort I'm able to apply to the difficult task. It increases my tenacity.[60] The thought of these rewards will help me through the challenges I'm facing. Similarly, we will use rewards to motivate our children to do more of the things we want them to (e.g., "tidy your bedroom and you'll get your allowance/we'll watch a film or play a game together").

Rewards are critical in decision-making, because they influence our motivation to do things and therefore our opportunity for learning (e.g., if I get a job at the local shop, I'll get paid, which means I can buy my own clothes/go out with my friends; in the process I develop the knowledge and skills of working in a shop. I commit to getting up early, getting to work on time, respecting the manager and customers—because I want to get paid this month).

What happens when we get less reward?

When we get less reward out of things, we start to FEEL-LOW; we tend to stop doing the things that matter, and so—we get less out of life. This sets up a vicious cycle of low mood, which can lead to the low-mood trap (see the illustration below). A simple, but effective, approach to managing this is engaging in more activities that are enjoyable, important, or meaningful. Research shows that by doing this (behavioral activation), it's possible to break free from the low-mood trap and start to feel better.[61] As you can see in the diagram, doing more of what matters helps you feel better and helps you get more out of life. It's the feel-good cycle.

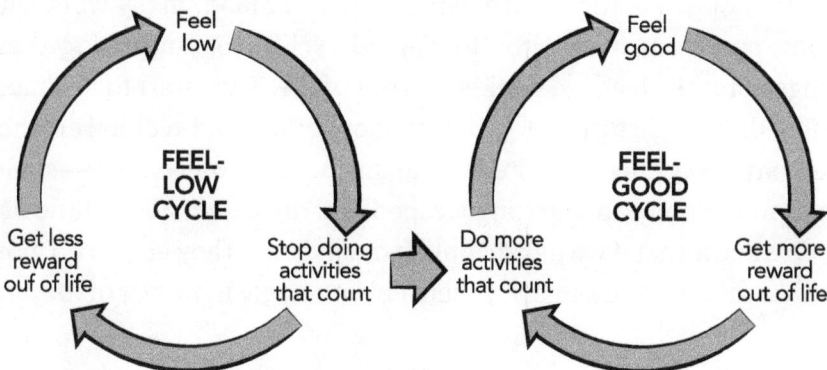

Feel low

FEEL-LOW CYCLE

Get less reward ouf of life

Stop doing activities that count

Do more activities that count

Feel good

FEEL-GOOD CYCLE

Get more reward out of life

As described by Laura Pass and Shirley Reynolds, behavioral activation (a psychological treatment for depression) is all about doing more activities that are helpful and important, and doing fewer activities that are unhelpful. It's powerful because **doing things differently leads to thinking and feeling differently.** We tend to think that we have to work on our thoughts and feelings first, but research tells us it's the doing that can have the biggest impact on our thinking (reflect back on chapter 9 where we explored acts of courage—brave behaviors lead to confidence and new skills).

Working out what's important

A lot of the work I do with young people when they are feeling low or depressed is helping them work out what's most important to them (this is an essential element of behavioral activation therapy). It's vital that when doing this the focus is on what's important to them, not to their parent, their teacher, siblings, or friends. Go back to the values activity in chapter 6 and identify the things that are important to them in three key areas: achievement (e.g., education/work, hopes and dreams for the future); what they enjoy and have fun doing (e.g., hobbies, how they look after themselves), and their relationships (e.g., family, friends, and romantic relationships).

When we, as parents, explore this more deeply with our children, we may find that the things that are most important to them, such as spending time with friends, doing well at school/sports, are those they've stopped doing since experiencing low mood. In my work with young people, I explain the low-mood cycle. Stopping doing these things naturally leads to getting less out of life. They start to feel more fatigued, have disturbed sleep, lose motivation, and feel lower; then they have less energy, more hopelessness, and do even less—sometimes to the point that getting washed and dressed can feel difficult.

We know that if we help people (whatever age they are) to do more of what matters to them, they then feel better, get more out of life, and are more inclined to do what matters to them and the cycle shifts toward feeling good (behavioral activation has a big evidence base).

It's vital that we don't wait until our mood improves, or our energy increases before we do things that count. What lots of young people I work with are waiting for when they experience low mood is to feel good enough, motivated enough, and energized enough to do the things that are important to them—they believe that it's only when they get to that point that they can start doing these things. Action creates motivation. Research suggests if we force ourselves to do these things, especially if we understand the rationale, then we start to feel better. As I observed with my children in the pandemic, going to key-worker school and changing their daily activities led to an improvement in mood.

Activity planning

What we do, where and with whom we spend our time can have a big impact on mood. A crucial aspect of behavioral activation therapy is to establish a connection between mood and activity, which can be achieved effectively by keeping a daily diary. As parents, we can help our child make the link between their current activities and their mood, and encourage them to do more activities that they will find meaningful and/or enjoyable. The activity diary below can be used to help your child log what they are currently doing with their time (everything from sleeping and scrolling on their phones to lying on their bed and daydreaming). Once this has been logged over a few days, you can begin to make the link between their mood and how they are spending their time. You can then think collaboratively about how they can include more things in their day that will give them a stronger sense of achievement, closeness and/or joy. As a parent, you can support them in overcoming any hurdles to doing these activities. They can continue to keep a diary, and this will show which activities are linked to an improvement in mood. Follow the instructions below for how to complete this task, and refer to the already completed example as a guide (this type of activity monitoring and planning activities is part of the behavioral activation approach). If your child is reluctant to engage with you doing this with pen and paper, signpost them to the free app Move Mood, which covers this approach digitally.

ACTIVITY BOX

Setting up the task

1. As the parent, complete this activity for yourself first, to help you get a feel for it. Then, sit down with your child (12+) and work together to complete the diary, using the worksheet in the resource pack as a guide (page 235 covers how to do this activity with under-twelves).

The task

2. Help them fill out as much detail as they are willing to share. Refer to a recent time (ideally the day before, or that day) to help them understand the task.
3. With your child, write down any activities they do (no matter how small or boring they seem) in the boxes below.
4. For each activity, support them to rate them out of ten for:
   a. Achievement—0 = Didn't achieve anything, to 10 = Huge achievement
   b. Closeness—0 = No closeness (on my own), to 10 = Felt very close to another
   c. Enjoyment—0 = No enjoyment, to 10 = Really enjoyed it
5. Once they've completed the log of the day with you, ask them to rate their overall mood for the day out of 10 (0 = Really low, unhappy, to 10 = Really upbeat, happy).
6. Ask your child if they think their mood is linked to the activities they are doing and what their scores are for achievement, closeness, and enjoyment.
7. Once they understand the task, ask them to complete the diary for two different days (one school, one not) the following week.

8. Once they've completed the task, look through the diary together and explore the parts of the day their mood seemed to be lowest and highest. See if there are any links to the activities they are doing or not doing.

9. Help your child think about alternative activities that would be meaningful or important to them. The Wellbeing Abacus may help guide you. Write a list of things they currently or used to enjoy. Consider how they might try to include some of these activities in the following days.

10. Think about how you can support your child to access these activities to reduce barriers, such as giving them a lift to a friend's house or inviting them to come out on a dog walk with you (with the added benefit of a hot chocolate, cold drink, or snack).

11. Continue to use the diary sheet to log the activities over the coming weeks. Your child should make the link that the more activities they do that are important to them, that give them either a sense of achievement, enjoyment, and/or closeness to valued others, the better their mood will be.

Day/ Time	Activity	Achievement	Closeness	Enjoyment
Wed 08:00	Breakfast with parents and sister	0	4	4
Wed 08:30	Bus to school, sat on my own	0	0	2
Wed 09:30	Math lesson. Zoned out	2	0	2
Wed 10:30	Break, went to library with two friends	5	7	7
Wed 11:30	Art lesson—completed sculpture	7	1	6
Sat 11:00	Spent two hours on Instagram/YouTube	0	2	2
Sat 13:00	Helped sister make brownies	5	6	6

Day/ Time	Activity	Achievement	Closeness	Enjoyment
Sat 15:00	Made a creative video, posted online; got lots of positive feedback from friends	6	6	7
Sat 18:00	Mom complained I hadn't tidied up. In my room on my own, lay on bed, stared at ceiling	0	0	0

Daily mood score: 0 = Really low, unhappy, to 10 = Upbeat, happy
Wed = 5; Sat at 3 p.m. = 7, Sat at 10 p.m. = 3

CASE STUDY

Charlie's Story (Part 2)

Charlie completed the activity log for two days. On the day he was going to school, he noticed that some of the activities on the list were scoring low for achievement, closeness, and enjoyment. At break, he spent time with a couple of friends in the library and his scores were higher for closeness, achievement, and enjoyment. He also noticed in the lesson he was able to engage, he worked better and felt a stronger sense of achievement and enjoyment. On a non-school day, Charlie noticed that spending time in his bedroom passively scrolling on social media or lying on his bed not doing anything were getting low scores across the board. However, when he had been engaging online with creating content, he found he had higher scores across all three. He also noticed, if he had time with his family relaxing or doing an activity like cooking, he felt more enjoyment and closeness compared to when he was with family and his parents were pressuring him to join in on an activity he was not interested in. His low mood score was largely consistent on Wednesday (a school day), but for Saturday, when he was at home, he noticed it was higher after the activities in the day, but dipped after a disagreement with his mom.

Doing this activity is helpful in a number of ways. Firstly, young people start to notice that their low mood isn't coming out of nowhere. Instead, it tends to be linked to what they are doing and with whom. Often it's triggered by interpersonal difficulties or conflict. Secondly, making the link between activities that reduce feelings of wellbeing and those that boost it helps young people to get better at regulating their activities when they start to notice feeling low. For example, in the following week when Charlie was beginning to feel low, he asked his friends if they could meet at lunchtime at school. At home, he recognized that withdrawing and being on his own doing nothing or going on Instagram made him feel worse. Instead, he started to notice feeling low and was then able to think: what important activity can I do to give me a boost?

A note on younger children

Earlier I mentioned my nine-year-old son who was struggling with low mood and the impact this was having on what he wanted to spend his time doing (on his screen) and his energy levels (lying around). He was not old enough for us to be able to do the activity diary together. However, I could spend time with him discussing the things he enjoys doing the most (holding in mind the achievement, closeness, and enjoyment areas). We talked about what was important to him and how he could get more time in the week to do these things. As a parent, I was able to observe and log how he was spending his time so that I could start to make some of the links between his activities and his better days. Again, the Wellbeing Abacus might be a useful guide and visual tool to shape these conversations.

For him, football is a big pleasure. He had stopped playing on Saturday with his team as he felt it was too much pressure. Instead, he and I looked for other ways he could play football in a more relaxed setting, finding an after-school club on a Wednesday. Although this seemed counterintuitive, as I was suggesting he spend more time at school—when he wanted to be there less—he joined the club and, on those days, came home with more energy and enthusiasm. I was also able to take him to another sports club outside of school during the week, which he really enjoyed. This had the added benefit of reducing his screen time (which we had worked out was not helping his mood). Most nights we built in a short period at bedtime (ten minutes or so) where we would play a simple game and he would read to me. Spending time together seemed to anchor his day and provide him with a safe space to share any worries. Within a couple of weeks, his energy and confidence had come back, he'd rejoined his Saturday team and was less irritable and withdrawn.

While he was at school I had less influence on how he spent his time, so to resolve this I asked for some support. Together—the class teacher, my son and I—thought about the boredom he was feeling there. My son likes additional responsibility and being challenged, so we agreed him having more opportunities for responsibility would be helpful. He applied to work in the library and his teacher gave him more tasks in lessons to support the classroom activities. Although he still was clear he would rather not be at school, this approach helped him find school more stimulating and improved his engagement.

This is a good example of how, by tuning into low feelings and using them to work out what was important to my son, we were able to make some simple changes that overcame the difficulties and gave him more opportunities to increase the things he found rewarding (see chapter 6). Consequently, with this support he was able to break free from the low-mood trap and spend his time doing more of what was important to him, which meant his mood and energy levels improved and I saw my fun-loving son return.

Helping our children access rewards

How can we help our young people access rewards (e.g., the things that are important in their life)? Sometimes this can feel easier with younger children, as often we will be the source of their rewards. Giving them our focus, praise, interest, and attention can support and motivate them to feel better about themselves and their world. Our time is often the biggest gift of all. We can set aside small amounts of time (simply ten to twenty minutes) to be alongside our child/adolescent and be present in their world (see page 111 for suggestions on how to do this).

With teenagers this can be more difficult, as they can be inclined to push us away and possibly want more time away from us (whether they are struggling with low mood or not). They also may be responsive to a different range of rewards because of the brain changes described on page 285. Here, we can help them consider what rewards they might value and remove the barriers to things they might not have the energy to do but are important to them, such as dropping them off at a friend's house—giving them practical support to access activities they enjoy.

> ### ☁ Reflection Box
>
> Think about your child. What is important to them? What are the rewards they care about and respond to? How can you provide them with more opportunities to access these rewards?
>
> Ideally by completing more activities that are important to them, they will increase the range of rewards they are experiencing. But it might help to think about really tangible rewards, particularly in the early days. Some ideas parents have shared with me include getting a takeaway, going to the cinema, seeing friends, going shopping, games and money. One of the most powerful rewards for most young people is more uninterrupted time with you. Playing a game or watching a favorite program of their choice together are often firm favorites. See page 111 for more ideas, particularly with adolescents. Remember the Wellbeing Abacus and note that activities that support these areas are likely to be most rewarding.

In chapter 14, I talk about the concept of "manager to coach." Essentially, this is moving toward a more collaborative approach with our teenagers, giving them more choice and guiding, rather than instructing. When I'm working with families, we tend to explore how parents can use this "coaching" approach while providing more opportunities for their adolescent to do more of what's important to them. This is particularly valuable, as we want to support the development of their identity and sense of autonomy. Doing this often involves compromise for us as parents, and we may need to let go of control (and criticism) of some aspects of family life.

For example, if we want to engage our adolescent in the evening meal, we may need to let them choose what they might like to cook for dinner, or allow them to cook in the kitchen, doing things their way as they learn to develop the skills. (It could be messier than we might like and we may need to stay clear of the kitchen to allow them to develop some autonomy!) You know your individual teenager—getting the balance of giving freedom, but also setting them up so they are more likely to succeed so they build confidence is also important (e.g., don't expect a Michelin-star meal or an immaculate kitchen at their first attempt). Perhaps if we were ordering a takeaway, we could encourage them to take more responsibility by letting them place the order for the family. We may have to privilege and encourage some of the things they value, as we support them in developing their identity (e.g., letting them play their music in the kitchen/car, showing an interest in their online world or friendship group without passing judgment).

Other top tips, to support access to rewards

* Encourage your child to pair up something they enjoy with a boring or less-desired task (e.g., meeting up with a friend to do schoolwork/revision together, listening to a podcast while doing the washing up).

* Find ways to celebrate your child's small achievements, whether that is verbal praise (e.g., "I feel so proud you tidied your room this morning. I know how hard you've found it with your energy levels, thank you.") or more concrete rewards (e.g., "Well done for making it into school this week on time. I got your favorite snack to acknowledge the effort you put into this.").

* Provide more opportunities for your young person to engage in flow activities (see page 73) and to develop a sense of mastery, especially in creative or sports activities (which are great at helping to balance both the dopamine and the stress-response seesaw).

* Rewards are less rewarding if they become predictable. Unexpected rewards have the biggest boost on our dopamine system. Consider how your young person can access novelty and how you can surprise them with unexpected positive affirmation.

* As described in chapter 3, ensure your child's rewards are not all linked to digital technology. Some research suggests young people struggling with low mood spend more time on their digital devices, which can interrupt important elements that contribute to wellbeing. Return to page 67 to consider how their use of digital technology might be impacting sleep, eating and physical activity. Consider also the range of in-person versus digital social contacts and activities they are having, which could contribute to a reduction in access to more edifying rewards (page 61).

* Build in an acts-of-kindness activity (page 36), as this has been shown to improve feelings of both anxiety and depression.

Unhooking from unhelpful thoughts

Chapter 8 explores in more detail the impact of our thoughts on how we feel and how to break free from worry and negative thinking patterns. This is particularly relevant for low mood. A big component that drives low mood is rumination (unwanted thoughts getting stuck on a loop in our minds). Rumination is unhelpful, as it triggers the stress response and inhibits the production of dopamine (see page 222). Helping our children unhook from unhelpful thoughts and rumination is therefore a key area to support as a parent.

When your child is struggling with low mood, the narrative in their head is often articulated to us as parents as, "There's no point," "Everything is terrible," and/or "I'm always useless." The additional challenge we face is that in adolescence, regardless of whether a young person is struggling with low mood or not, they are likely to have a negativity bias toward anything that we're going to say as adults. This makes it hard to have helpful conversations when our young person may make these statements. We're likely to jump in with, "No, that isn't true," or "What do you mean?," which moves us away from connecting with our child. Chapter 13 gives you some communication tools to help with this dilemma. Before we get into these, I'll share some ideas on how you can support your child or adolescent unhook from negative thoughts.

You might know from personal experience what it feels like to get stuck in negative thoughts, how depleting and draining it is. In these moments, the thoughts feel so real that it's really tough to create that distance between you and your thoughts, often because these thoughts are about things that you deeply care about.

Top Tips: Creating distance between you and your thoughts (share and model with your young person)

▶ **Label it**. *It's just a thought—it doesn't mean it's real.* Remind yourself that thoughts are not facts. Often a feeling of dread can give us a sense that this feeling is a premonition that something bad is going to happen. Reminding ourselves that thoughts are just ideas and they do not predict the future is important (see "If I keep worrying, bad things won't happen" on page 173).

▶ **Let the thoughts come and go**. Noticing a thought and letting it come and go (see "drop the rope" on page 181) is a helpful way to reduce rumination. This activity helps us get used to letting thoughts come and go rather than them overwhelming or overpowering us. It can be as simple as saying to ourselves, "Ah—I notice I'm having that thought again, thank you, brain, for trying to look out for me, but I don't think I need to get stuck with this. I'm going to move my attention to something else." The practice of mindfulness helps by encouraging us to learn to move our attention to something else, even if we're feeling overwhelmed.

▶ **Take the power out of the thought**. Repeating the thought to ourselves in a silly voice (e.g., a Donald Duck voice) might make us laugh. Often, humor can help dissipate the power of the thought. Sharing the thought with another person can be sufficient to take the power out of the thought and get some feedback on its validity. Many young people I work with worry about their worrying thoughts, their content and what it means about them. Sharing them with another, understanding they may be fairly normal in the circumstances, and getting a wise viewpoint has often helped the thought lose its power or stopped it growing in magnitude.

▶ **Leave it alone or refocus on something else**. Lots of young people get stuck in their bedrooms, often lying on their bed in the dark, perhaps scrolling through social media—marinating in their distressing thoughts. I always suggest to young people that in these moments they need to move to doing something else: get up, leave their room, and take some kind of helpful action. Mel Robbins talks about the five-second rule.[62] Essentially, when you're not feeling like doing something important or required, by simply counting down from five, four, three, two, one, to "Go!" and physically moving toward the activity at "Go!," you can overpower procrastination and lack of action (e.g., "I'm feeling worse; lying on my bed is not helping. I need to move downstairs and be with others. I'm going to count backwards and move toward my bedroom door. Five, four, three, two, one . . . Go!").

The most important job as a parent: Providing opportunities for connection

One of the critical things we can do as a parent is ensure our children know we're available for them when they need us and that we will try our best to not minimize or overreact when they tell us how difficult they are finding things. As talked about in chapter 6, if our children can see that we can cope with their distress, in the moments they share what's going on for them, they will feel confident that we're ready and able to support them when they reach out. Our response to them in these moments is going to determine how willing they feel to return to us in the future when things are difficult. In part 2, we explored how we can respond to our children in such moments and chapter 13 will build on this, providing key communication tips to help us not only respond well to our children when they ask for help, but also how to reach out to them when they are struggling to ask for support.

SUMMARY

→ How we spend our time impacts our mood and activity levels.

→ Rewards are an important part of life: they motivate us, help us build skills and a sense of mastery as well as improve our mood.

→ When we feel low, we tend to do less of what's important to us, meaning we get less reward from life and feel lower—this is the low-mood cycle.

→ By doing more of what's important to us on a daily basis, we get more reward from life and start to feel better—this is the feel-good cycle.

→ Working out what's important to a young person is a key first step to working out what activities they can do more of and what unhelpful activities they can do less of.

→ As a parent, you can support your child by providing more opportunities to do what's important to them and increase their access to rewards.

→ Negative thoughts can impact our child's motivation to do what's important to them. We can help them unhook from these thoughts by encouraging them to label the thoughts, let them go, take the power out of them, and focus on something else.

→ The way we communicate and respond when our children face difficulties can impact how comfortable they feel seeking our support during tough times.

Chapter 12
Self-harm

I gently touch my daughter's arm, an affectionate gesture. A jolt of confusion hits me as instead of soft flesh, I feel hard scabs. I turn her arm toward me and see the angry marks; precise, inch-long cuts. Earlier in the week I had commented in the car on some marks on her hand, which looked out of place, red-raw scratches among pen marks. A game she had been playing with her friends, she said. I wanted to believe her. I did believe her. But my brain is now struggling to ignore what this might be. I look at her and she realizes I've noticed. She pulls her arm away, moves quickly and locks herself in the bathroom. "I don't want to talk about it; leave me alone!" she cries through the door. I follow her and stand outside the door, calling her name gently. "Emily, it's OK, I'm not angry. You can talk to me." Inside and out, I'm shaking. Powerless, afraid, angry. I just don't understand. Why? Why would my daughter, so fierce and brave, so seemingly capable, hurt herself like this? The door stays firmly shut. At a loss, I return to my bedroom. I feel sick inside. Scared. What does this mean? What do I do? How do I help? Is it my fault? I pick up my phone. I want to reach out to some-one—but who? This is a private thing—my daughter's thing. What if others judge her, write her off—think it's attention-seeking, or she's mentally ill? What if they blame me as her parent? The stigma, the judgment, the awkwardness of others. I can't face it. I put my phone down. I hear my daughter go to her bedroom. I pick my phone back up. I send her a message: I love you. I want to help. I see she's online, the two blue ticks. Then she's typing. I hold my breath.

Account from a parent

What is self-harm?

Self-harm is when someone deliberately harms themselves. This could be through a physical injury (e.g., self-hitting, banging, wound-picking, scratching, cutting, pinching, self-biting, pulling hair), self-poisoning (e.g., taking too much medication) or another method of harming the body (e.g., restricting eating, over-exercise, alcohol, drugs). Across the world, about 17 percent of adolescents (aged twelve to eighteen) deliberately injure themselves each year. There are concerns that more and more young people are self-harming, with a 68 percent increase in incidents of self-harm reported in girls aged thirteen to sixteen years old from 2011 to 2014.[63]

Any parent reading these statistics is likely to feel concerned. As a parent who knows or suspects their child has self-harmed, your feelings are likely to be strong and reflect that of the parent in the opening paragraph: shock, distress, anger, sadness, helplessness and the overwhelming questions: "Why?" and "What do I do?" Before you attempt to look for the answers, take a deep breath. Wrap your arms around yourself and give yourself a hug. This is a difficult topic. Self-harm is an important message that your child is not coping with some of the challenges in their life. Find reassurance in knowing that you can help by providing your support and if required enabling your child to get additional support. They do not need to be alone with this, and neither do you.

A note on this chapter

There are many excellent resources available for parents on self-harm, which cover the topic in lots of detail. There is simply not enough room in this book to cover it all, and it would be a mistake to try to do so. I've written this chapter, not with the hope of replicating this information, but instead focusing on the elements I feel are most pertinent, based on the conversations I've had with parents and young people. Please use the additional resources (signposted to in the Further Resources section) if this is a topic relevant to you, as there are elements I will not cover here (e.g., managing injuries, alternatives to self-harm).

Indicators of self-harming behaviors

These signs do not necessarily mean your child is self-harming. If more of these items are ticked, then the probability of self-harm is higher. Take notice of:

* clothing—changes in clothing to cover parts of the body (long sleeves even in warm weather), blood stains on clothing (including bedding/towels), not wanting to join in activities that involve less cover from clothing;

* cuts, bruises, scratches, and/or burns that appear and have scant explanation;

* sharp or cutting objects among a person's belongings (e.g., pencil sharpener blades, compass, razor blades);

* low or fluctuating mood, increased irritability:
  * becoming withdrawn, isolated;
  * low self-esteem and self-blame;
  * changes in eating/sleeping;
  * poor performance at school/work;
  * loss of interest in favorite activities.

Why self-harm?

If a young person has harmed themselves, they are likely to be experiencing some difficulties in their life that they are struggling to cope with. These difficulties may lead to strong, unpleasant thoughts and feelings which can become overwhelming. If a young person does not have other ways to cope, they may discover self-harm can be a quick way to relieve those feelings, as a form of self-soothing. When parents grasp this idea, it can come as a relief that the self-harm has a function beyond damage to the body.

Feeling too much

Research shows that just before self-harming, people experience high levels of emotional distress, and immediately afterward, this distress significantly reduces.[64] Self-harm, therefore, is a powerful way to help regulate emotions and reduce distress.

Feeling too little

Self-harm can help when someone feels overwhelmed to the point they feel nothing at all (numb) or detached from themselves (dissociate). The act of self-harm (experiencing physical pain) can help a person reconnect to feeling something, even if it's pain, making them feel more alive and real.

Young people say self-harm helps:

* reduce negative feelings;
* relieve tension or a sense of pressure;
* provide a distraction from negative thoughts;
* increase positive feelings, including feeling calmer;
* give a sense of control over the problem or feelings;
* act as a form of self-punishment when feeling bad about themselves.

Although self-harm may create initial feelings of relief, these tend to be followed by feelings of guilt and shame, which can add to an overall sense of distress, perpetuating the self-harm cycle.

Understanding that self-harm is an expression of personal distress provides us with various ways to help our child:

1. We can consider what's causing the distress for our child and help resolve the situation or find ways of supporting our child to manage it.
2. We can support our child to learn healthier ways to relieve their distress, including encouraging them to share their distress

with us (and/or another trusted adult) so they can experience the loving reassurance that they are not alone.

What could be causing distress?

When self-harm shows up, understanding what's creating the distress is very important. Look in the activity box below at the issues associated with self-harm. What might be happening in your child's life that could be contributing to their distress? Note the issues you recognize that might be impacting your child. Consider any other issues unique to your child.

ACTIVITY BOX

Relationship difficulties	Gender identity	Anxiety	Struggling academically
Bereavement	School pressures	Parental conflict	Discrimination
Disability	Emotional abuse	Physical abuse	Not going to school
Chronic physical illness	Conflict with parents	Neglect	Drug/alcohol use
Parental mental health	Worries about money	Bullying	Lack of close friends
Exposure to self-harm (friends/family)	Media and internet influence	Low mood	Sexual identity

There are things that can help protect children from self-harm: understanding parents, having close friends, and doing well at school.

Look at the following box to think about the areas where your child may be struggling: in their home, school, and/or with friends. What practical and emotional support might your child need in each area to help with the distress? I have given some examples. If you feel like you don't know what your child is struggling with, don't be afraid to start a conversation with them using the tools on pages 104–106.

	Home	School	Friends
What is my child finding hard/ difficult in this area?	Spending too much time alone.	Struggling with math lessons.	Feeling different and isolated.
How can I support my child emotionally? Who else can help?	Provide safe space to talk. Include trusted family members.	Validate feelings and reassure support can help. Teacher or tutor.	Validate feelings. School staff, youth club, family, or friend.
What practical things can help?	Spend 1-to-1 time doing an activity of their choice 15 mins a day.	Speak to school. Support study time, provide encouragement and comfort.	Reduce barriers to meeting up with friends. Support joining a community of like-minded young people.

Often when a young person self-harms, the injury can grab the focus of everyone's attention, which distracts us from addressing the adolescent's underlying needs. Expecting a young person to stop feeling such intense feelings or stop self-harming if their needs are not met is unfair on them. Imagine someone is sweating because they have a temperature—the sweating is a symptom of the temperature. Understanding why the person has a temperature is the key to understanding how to treat the temperature, at which point the sweating stops. Take a look at James's story below, but take care, as this may bring up strong feelings for you. Read it when you feel well-resourced: right time, right place, right pace.

- -

CASE STUDY

James's Story

James is a fourteen-year-old boy who lives at home with his mom. He has never had contact with his dad. His mom works long hours on a shift pattern and gets home at 10 p.m., well after James has returned from school. Money is and always has been tight. James feels he is very self-sufficient. He sees school as a good place to be and often stays at after-school clubs to reduce the amount of time he's at home on his own. When he gets back, he tends to walk the dog, have a snack and watch something/game until his mom gets home. Mom makes dinner and they eat together late. They both go to sleep after midnight. James notices that his life is different from his friends', but he has always coped. However, a month ago, his dog died. He was devastated. Coming home after school, he felt moments of total aloneness and was so overwhelmed with a mixture of sadness and emptiness that he felt he might die from the pain. He discovered if he banged his head hard, it would distract and relieve him. Feeling a sense of calm, he would then go to sleep until his mom got home. Having slept earlier in the evening meant it was difficult to sleep at night. He would lie awake with dark thoughts about his life and the point of it all. Head-banging turned to cutting after he looked it up on the internet and saw images. He would think of cutting as a safety blanket, something he almost looked forward to and part of the routine of managing when he came home. He got into a pattern where school, self-harm and sleep felt like the only places he could escape from his intense sadness and sense of hopelessness. One day, as school finished, he went to his tutor and said he was worried if he went home that night he would kill himself. He didn't want to worry his mom by telling her how he was feeling—she had enough on her plate—but he couldn't face another evening of the pattern he was in. He was ashamed, afraid and lonely. He didn't want to die, but he didn't know how to escape the place he found himself in, where he didn't want to be anymore.

- -

Reading James's story, how does it make you feel? What does your instinct tell you about James's needs? What makes it hard for James to get what he needs? If we think of James's self-harm and thoughts of dying as the sweating (symptoms), then we should consider the underlying temperature (the cause) as feelings of grief and sadness over the death of his dog, loneliness and isolation from having limited time with his mom and long stints alone. By understanding his self-harm in this sense, we can focus on finding the most helpful ways to support James both practically and emotionally. Let's now think about the first step to helping a child when we become aware of their self-harm or distress.

What to do

When we discover a child has self-harmed, whether through them telling/showing us, or it coming to our attention another way, it gives rise to an immediate emotional response in us. Our own stress response kicks in, and we might go into fight (get upset, angry), flight (avoid the conversation, distract with something else), or freeze mode (shut down and find it hard to provide any response).

Imagine the worst thing you've ever done or the thoughts you've had that you feel most ashamed and guilty about. Picture these thoughts/actions being on your arm, exposed, for another person to see. When the other person looks at the thing of which you're most deeply ashamed, and then looks up at you, what do you want to do? What do you need from them in that moment?

Both Emily's—the girl from the beginning of the chapter—and James's vulnerability was extremely high when their distress (self-harm marks, thoughts of wanting to die) was revealed to others. In those moments, how the other person responded would either soothe and contain them—or cause more pain. As described in chapter 5, providing the response a child needs at this time involves the four stages: notice, connect, validate and collaborate.

Notice

Paying attention to your own feelings and finding a way to help yourself feel more grounded or calm (taking deep breaths) can help you focus on how to support your child. Emily's mom's emotions were so strong in the moment of realization that it was hard to provide an immediate, soothing response. Emily ran away to hide her vulnerability and shame. If you're reading this as a parent who has had this experience, you may be able to recognize a similar scenario that has played out for you. The important thing for Emily and her mom was that even though her mom was shocked and couldn't hide her reaction, she took a pause, a deep breath, and came back to her daughter quickly enough to share with her that she was not cross, but that she loved her. She wanted to find a way to help. She respected her daughter's need for space but remained available and in touch, in a way that the daughter could engage with.

Connection and validation

Finding ways to connect to your child so that they can sense your presence and experience it as calming and reassuring is powerful in immediately reducing their distress. Being able to connect to their distress without being overwhelmed by it and validating their feelings is a soothing balm that can help your child feel less alone, less afraid of rejection, and shows them their feelings are real and important. This helps them to understand that despite it being difficult, hope is not lost, and there are things that can help. Remember, often it's not what we say, but how we say it, that counts. In these moments, your child needs you as their parent, not an expert.

Finding what works for your child

Young people often tell me that they are happy for parents or adults to check with them the best way to communicate and also other ways of communicating love and care. Some young people find touch reassuring when they are feeling distressed; others don't want to be touched or held. Don't be afraid to warmly ask your young person what their preferences are so that you can respect them. "I really want to help—what feels most helpful to you? Talking or messaging? Would you like me to hold your hand/hug you?"

Initially, when our child needs to reach out for help, they might not want to talk with us face to face. They may prefer to share what's happening for them through texting or writing a letter. Our child's preferences (not speaking face to face, not wanting physical connection) can feel so hard as a parent—so rejecting and impersonal—but sometimes texting, writing, and communicating in these ways can feel less intense and help a young person manage their vulnerability enough that they can open up to you. The key is using this medium as you would hope to in person: with warmth, understanding, conveying your love and validation. It's a gateway to communicating better face to face and reconnecting with your child, to building trust and moving toward your child being able to be more vulnerable in person. With some parents and young people, sending an empty text message or a text message with a particular word or symbol (something symbolic to them that you've worked out together) can be a way a young person lets their parent know they need the parent to be present and provide support. This presence might likely mean coming alongside your child and doing an activity together so they do not feel isolated. They may then use this time to open up to you (remember the tips on page 111).

Collaboration

Once our children feel understood, we can then think with them about practical ways that we can help. Together, we can explore: (1) how to create increased parental emotional availability and support from other trusted adults over the coming weeks and months to help your child feel cared for (see page 295 for ideas on this); and (2) practical ways to reduce the stressors in their lives that might be contributing to their distress (at the right time, this could involve using the problem-solving approach on page 175).

Getting more help

Young people who self-harm find getting support from those people already in their lives is very helpful (including family, friends and other members of the community: school, youth clubs, faith communities). Some young people will need additional support from a professional. I would recommend speaking with your child's school, school nurse, or family doctor, to enable them to help you and your child get the correct support in place if they consider more assistance is needed. Self-harm can have a big impact, not just on the child and their parents, but also on other family members (siblings). Many parents benefit from having access to a parental support group, as it can be difficult for friends and family to understand the unique concerns that self-harm brings. I always advocate increasing your and your family's support network when struggling with your child's mental health; it can be a huge relief to everyone to feel understood and less alone. Any adult responding to a child in distress or who has self-harmed can use the principles in the box below.

Useful phrases to support a young person in distress

* "Thank you for coming to me—I want to help. Things sound really tough right now. I'm wondering if we should move to a quieter place. Are you happy to go to another room?"

* "It sounds like you have a lot going on for you right now. Thank you for telling me. What would be helpful for me to know?"

* "Oh dear, that sounds sad. I imagine that must have really hurt your feelings."

* "I can understand that. You don't have to be alone with this. There are things that we can think about together to help. We can find a way through this together."

* "Thank you for being brave and telling me how you're feeling. I understand it's not easy. I'm so proud of you."

Do:	Don't:
• Right time, right place, right pace (page 111).	• Focus on the impact on you as the parent/adult.
• Express warmth and non-judgment.	• Tell or ask the young person not to self-harm again.
• Explain that you're not angry, but your voice and face might seem worried, because you deeply care.	• Communicate in a way that works for you, but not for them.
• Help them feel like you want to find ways to help and/or enable help.	• Make the young person feel like they've done something bad or are in trouble.
• Understand and validate feelings.	
• Be curious about what they are finding hard in their life.	• Only give care to a young person around the self-harm incidents.
Once you've done all of this:	• Assume that the young person wants to end their life.
• Find a way to make a plan together so they don't have to feel so alone.	

Suicidal thoughts

It's natural to be concerned that your child might be experiencing suicidal thoughts if they are deliberately hurting themselves. Many young people will self-harm without suicidal thoughts. Others will have suicidal thoughts without self-harm. Regardless of the self-harm, the idea or knowledge of your child not wanting to be alive, and potentially acting on this, is one of the most terrifying fears a parent can have. Hence, asking your child about their suicidal thoughts can feel so daunting.

For many people who end or attempt to end their life, the stigma around asking for help often prevents them from reaching out and getting the necessary support. As parents, we have an important role to play in observing changes in our child's behavior that might suggest our child is struggling with their mental health and asking them directly whether they are thinking about suicide. We can use the tools in this chapter to help us navigate compassionate and curious conversations with our young person, but if we have concerns, it's important that we ask clear, closed questions like, "Are you thinking about suicide/taking your own life/ending your life?"

It's a misconception that if we ask about suicide, we might put this thought into a young person's head or make them feel worse. If a young person is thinking about suicide, they will undoubtedly feel very alone with these thoughts. Being able to share these with someone safely can help them feel less alone and provides an opportunity to give that person the help they need to manage the crisis they are in.

A young person might be thinking about wanting to die or ending their life (suicidal ideation), but not have any plans or intent to do so. Some young people may be actively suicidal; they may have planned how they would end their life and intend to act on it.

Talking with our child directly about this concern can open up the opportunity to share if they do have thoughts or plans about ending their life. We're then able, after connecting with and validating their feelings, to think about how to help them stay safe and get access to more help for them.

The American Academy of Pediatrics has a suicide safety planning tool that professionals can use to support this conversation and help keep a young person safe. This would usually be shared with parents (see page 307). If your child is having suicidal thoughts, it's important they not only get support from you, but also from a professional. Contact your child's pediatrician and explain you need an urgent appointment and what the concerns are. Remove access to methods of self-harm (e.g., medication). If you're concerned you cannot keep your child safe, phone your local mental health crisis helpline. You'll find signposting to national helplines, crisis support, and some apps that your child might find helpful in the Further Resources at the end of this book (page 307).

The role of other supportive adults

Often parents are told that their child has self-harmed or might have thoughts about ending their life by another adult, usually a member of the school or medical staff. Often the child may have told a friend who then tells an adult. This can be deeply shocking and create feelings of shame in you as a parent ("Maybe it's my fault") and/or relief ("I'm so glad I'm not alone with this. Hopefully, this person can help"). In my line of work, I often have a conversation with the young person and then share the information about self-harm or suicidal thoughts with the parent. My observation is that children are worried and scared of hurting or adding to their parents' concerns. They feel ashamed, guilty, and anxious that their parent will be disappointed or reject them. At the same time, I see great relief. When I talk to that young person again, I see a huge burden lifted from them if their parent has provided a caring and loving response.

Try not to be hurt if your child tells someone else, not you. Because of their intense bond with you, they may find it hard to disclose. By not telling you how they feel, they may believe they are protecting you.

Often, they are aware that by telling another trusted adult, they are getting the information to you, so that you can help.

Your child will always need your love and support. However, having another trusted adult to talk to can allow them to feel less concerned about the impact of their feelings. When I talk with children, they trust it's my job to listen and help them. This takes away the anxiety that I might not be able to handle what they have to share.

Whether I'm working with a child and their family or not, I'm very clear. Your child needs your love and care, and the connection you offer them will help them manage the difficult times they are facing. Never doubt that. Sometimes you'll hold hope for your child. Sometimes you'll need the support of others to hold this hope for you and your child. But don't give up. Believe you can all get through this with the right help.

☀️ Self-harm Q&A

Q: Is my child doing this for attention?

A: Self-harming is not a way of seeking attention. It's often done in secret, with young people going to great lengths to hide it. Shame and guilt are feelings that go with self-harm, which makes it even more difficult to ask for help or talk about it. As a parent, it can feel confusing if your child has self-harmed in a very visible place (e.g., their hand) and gives the impression the self-harm is for attention. It's more likely that it's a way of communicating distress and the need for support from others.

Q: Does my child feel physical pain when they self-harm?

A: Yes. Although we do not yet fully understand the biology of self-harm, we know that endorphins play a role in

reinforcing self-harm as a way of managing distress.
Endorphins are how the body naturally downregulates pain,
both physical and social/emotional pain. After self-harming,
these endorphins may provide a natural high, helping to
relieve both the emotional and physical pain. For people who
repeatedly self-harm, some research shows their pain
thresholds can change, perhaps as they develop increased
tolerance.

Q: I've heard lots of young people are self-harming. Is my child
following a trend or trying to fit in?

A: Research is still trying to establish the social elements of self-
harm. A young person who self-harms will not do so simply to
fit in with a peer group. They will be self-harming to cope with
distress. It can be confusing for parents and school staff, as
young people who have friends who self-harm are more likely
to self-harm. This is what's called the "social contagion effect."
A distressed young person might initially try self-harm to cope
with their distress because they've been exposed to it in their
environment (seeing a close friend use this method, or through
viewing images and certain content online). It is important to
support your child to limit exposure to online self-harm
content.

Q: If I just ignore it, will it go away?

A: Some research suggests that many parents' first response to
their child's self-harming is to ignore it, in the hope that it will
pass. There is often the worry that paying attention to self-
harm might make it worse or reinforce it as a coping

mechanism. Recognizing your child's self-harm as a sign they are not coping and need help is important. Think about how you can increase your positive availability and encourage connection, so your child understands you're with them, not against them, and consider other support you can enlist.

SUMMARY

→ A child might hurt themselves to cope with emotional distress or communicate to others that they are distressed.

→ Self-harm can relieve distress temporarily, but increase it in the long term.

→ Understanding what's causing distress in a young person's life is an important first step in helping to support them.

→ Parents and trusted adults are a vital part of providing both practical and emotional support for a young person who is using self-harm as a way to cope with difficulties.

→ How we talk to young people about what's going on for them, as well as how we make ourselves available to support them, is critical: notice, connect, validate, collaborate.

→ Asking your child whether they are having thoughts about ending their life will not encourage them to take this action. Instead, it provides an opportunity for them to talk to you about their inner world and enables you to put safety plans in place if this is something they are considering.

→ Getting help from others for yourself and your child is important. Self-harm and the associated concerns about your child having thoughts of hurting themselves can create huge anxiety for families.

→ One of the most important things you can do is believe in yourself as an avenue of support for your child, but don't be afraid to seek additional support.

PART 5
Help

The secret to giving and getting

Chapter 13

Building strong relationships– communication hacks

All the young people I work with describe how difficult it is to talk to others about their thoughts and feelings when they are struggling, whether that is with friends or family. The sad reality is when our children's mental health deteriorates, so does their ability to reach out for support and communicate with others. However, connection and help from others is the most important contributor to wellbeing, so when children are least likely to ask for help and most likely to withdraw from us, it's likely then that they need us the most. As parents, this can be a painful and frustrating time for us, as our attempts to support and understand our children can result in the opposite response from them than we had hoped. Unintentionally, our responses to this may lead to further communication breakdown, isolation, and distress for both our children and us.

In this final section, we will explore how to communicate with our children when our relationships might be most tenuous, and how we can support them in getting the right help, at the right time, when we recognize their needs extend beyond what we can offer (head to the Further Resources section for more information on signposting).

Mood and relationships

The biggest predictor of overall happiness for all of us is our relationships. This is because our mood and our relationships are inter-connected—essentially, how we experience our relationships will impact how we feel (our mood). For example, an argument with a close friend may lead to feeling low, while having fun with a close friend may lead to feelings of happiness.

How we feel (our mood) influences what happens in our relationships. For example, feeling low and irritable may lead to more arguments, withdrawing from others, and relationship breakdown, while feeling positive and happy might lead to kindness, seeking out others, and improved relationships. The responses we get from these arguments or acts of kindness can reinforce our mood and, in turn, how well-connected we are to others.

This cycle (as shown in the diagram below) demonstrates that if we can improve our relationships, we can improve our mood and wellbeing. Teaching skills to do this is a vital part of empowering our children to manage the relationships in their life better, thus improving their wellbeing.

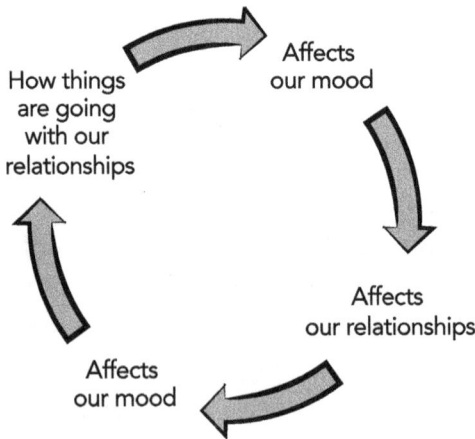

☁ Reflection Box

＊ Think of a recent scenario when you were in a bad mood, felt tired or stressed, and you acted differently toward another person (family member/friend) in a way that reflected this feeling. What happened next? (e.g., being in a bad mood led to feeling more annoyed, which led to an argument with, or withdrawal from, another person).

* Think of a recent scenario where difficulties in a relationship impacted your mood/stress levels (e.g., an argument with your partner has made you feel down).

* Think of a recent scenario where you've had a positive experience with others and it has impacted your mood (e.g., spending time with a close friend has made you feel happy and cared for).

* Which key people have the biggest impact on your mood? On your child's mood?

Emotions can make it difficult to communicate

My daughter and I seem to be having more arguments since she's turned thirteen (chapter 14 clarifies how adolescence may explain this!). Just the other day, she wanted me to take her to her friend's house immediately. I couldn't drop everything to do this. On hearing "no," she erupted into a rage and started telling me what a rubbish mom I was. This angered me, and I responded by telling her she was rude and inconsiderate. She then shouted (lid flipped now, page 91) that she wished she lived with her dad. My lid also flipped and I retorted, implying this wasn't a bad idea! She stormed off to her room where she spent the rest of the day. She didn't see her friend and felt angry about this. I'm guessing there was some guilt at saying the cruel things she had said to me as well. I spent the rest of the day feeling angry with myself for reacting, guilty that I hadn't stopped myself getting cross and wishing I had not said something that I didn't mean. I wondered if perhaps I should have been more willing to drop her at her friend's. We both spent the afternoon at separate ends of the house feeling terrible.

As described in Dialectical Behavioral Therapy (DBT), in our relationships we're often caught between the tension of:

* getting what we want and need from others;

* keeping (not destroying) the relationship; and

* maintaining self-respect (ensuring we're not compromising our values).

This complex combination of tasks often means our interactions with others are filled with emotions. These emotions can make it harder to communicate well and feel understood. As illustrated above, my daughter quickly became overwhelmed with anger, her lid flipped and what she said and did in those moments when her downstairs brain took over led to me quickly being overwhelmed by my own emotions (and doubts about being a good mom). With my lid flipped, our capacity for thinking and communicating well was destroyed.

Not only were we both left lower in mood for the remainder of the day, but my daughter did not get what she wanted (me to take her to her friend's), we experienced a rupture in our relationship (by saying hurtful things), and we both lost self-respect (felt bad about saying unkind things). For my daughter and I, this scenario offered the potential for:

* further conflict and deterioration in our relationship and decreased wellbeing; or

* learning, repairing, and developing the skills required to communicate in a more healthy and productive way.

By doing the latter, we could pave the way for resolving future conflict, building a stronger relationship with one another, and supporting the development of skills that can be used in other relationships.

As a parent, we know how difficult this task can be. Our attempts in the past may have led to a further escalation of distress and tension in the relationship, making us afraid to reach out to our child. If our young person is struggling with low mood they will be more irritable and sensitive to others, making it harder to communicate with them. Add to this our own stress levels and experiences of low mood, communicating well with those we care for can sometimes feel like an impossible task.

As outlined in part 2, how, when, and what we say can massively impact keeping our upstairs and downstairs brain connected, not only helping regulate our emotions, but also helping us communicate and build more positive relationships. The remainder of this chapter builds on this and outlines the practical things you can do to transform your communication with your child.

What you say and how you say it

It's not just what you say, but how you say it. Our tone of voice, non-verbal expressions and body language massively impact how the content of a message is received. This in turn influences the person's response, which can often determine the outcome of a conversation. My daughter in the above situation said, "Mom, can you take me to my friend's house now?" in an aggressive, loud, and demanding way. Her face looked cross and she intruded into my personal space to ensure I paid her full attention. The very same words, said in a calm and enquiring way, with my daughter smiling and her body language relaxed may have been enough for my response to have been, "let me see" rather than "no," leading to an entirely different outcome. The below skills from Dialectical Behavioral Therapy (DBT) are helpful in reminding us how to approach communicating with others to get the best outcome and reduce the probability of triggering the downstairs emotional brain, leading to a disconnect with the upstairs thinking brain.

GIVE Skills[65]

Gentle: Think tone of voice, respect.

Interested: Show you're listening by looking interested (e.g., nodding, good eye contact, and not interrupting).

Validate: Show you're trying to understand with warmth and curiously wondering aloud what you think might be going on for the other person (e.g., "I'm guessing this feels so upsetting because your friend is really important to you . . .").

Easy: Have a friendly posture, give enough personal space, with a kind tone of voice, be playful or use humor, if appropriate.

The GIVE principles are even more important when talking with teenagers as they are especially sensitive to being treated with respect. The physical changes they experience mean they are more attuned to social status. A little trick I use when talking with teenagers is imagining I'm talking to someone with the highest possible status—this can transform a conversation and lead to a more collaborative discussion.

The six communication hacks

In my work with adolescents, often the challenges they are facing in their relationships are having a huge impact on their lives. With emotions running high and a greater dependency on social relationships, the way that they are communicating with their world and the way their parents communicate with them can affect their wellbeing. I teach young people and their parents six communication hacks that are simple, but can profoundly change the dynamic in their relationships. These skills are from an evidence-based program called Interpersonal Psychotherapy-Adolescent Skills Training (IPT-AST) developed by Young, Mufson and Schueler (2016).[66] The idea is if you can teach adolescents effective communication and interpersonal problem-solving skills, you can support them to improve their relationships and prevent the development of depression. As part of the IPT-AST program young people are taught six communication skills: strike while the iron is cold; "I" statements; be specific; come with some solutions; put yourself in their shoes; and don't give up.[67] In my work with families I encourage parents and young people to develop their communication skills by using these six techniques. In doing so, family members learn how to develop the skills they need to negotiate the significant relationships in their lives, including the parent–child relationship. We'll shortly be exploring each of the skills and linking them back to Clara's story detailed below.

CASE STUDY

Clara's Story (Part 1)

Here we'll be following Clara, a seventeen-year-old girl who has been finding home and college life difficult recently.

Clara lives with her mom and her sister, who is fourteen. She tells me they are all arguing often. This means she wants to spend more time on her own in her bedroom or out with her friends. The only trouble is that her best friend has recently got a boyfriend and seems to want to spend most of her time with him or talking about him. Clara is feeling lonely and generally irritated with those around her. She finds it difficult to talk about this with her family and friends. When she tries, things seem to escalate into arguments and then she feels worse. She has begun to give up on communicating with others and feels herself relying more on social media and chat rooms to fill her time. Quite often the people in the chat rooms agree with how upset she must be feeling and give her advice about how she should dump her friend or have a go at her mom and sister. This advice seems to be sapping her energy and making her feel more distressed and alone. Clara wants to be able to spend more quality time with her mom and her best friend, but feels this is now not achievable. In the following section, we will use Clara's story to explain how Young et al.'s six communication hacks can help Clara get closer to her friends and family and improve her mood.

---

1 *Strike while the iron is cold*

Picking the right time to have a conversation is critical to the outcome of the conversation. Open and honest conversations are most likely to happen when we're feeling calm and not under pressure (see the window of tolerance on page 102). If either party in a conversation is feeling angry or distressed, it's more likely that you or the other person will not get the hoped-for outcome and very likely that either one of you may say something you later regret, like my daughter and I earlier in the chapter.

It's important that we're aware when we or the other person are not in the best frame of mind or context to have a difficult conversation. Learning the art of respectfully pausing the conversation and scheduling it for a better time (when you or the other person is **not** dealing with competing demands or feeling reactive) is an invaluable life skill. Also, if you have something you would like to talk about, asking the other person if they have time to talk and, if not, scheduling a better time to talk is a great tactic.

My children always seem to bring up a difficult issue at the worst time for me, typically when we're rushing out the door on our way to work and school. Often, they do not seem to be aware that I'm in a distracted frame of mind and therefore not likely to respond well to their question. Likewise, often I bring something up for my young person when they are not in the right frame of mind, and I'm unaware of this because they've not told me what's going on for them.

If the conversation has already started, *pause the conversation and organize for a better time.* Explain to your child, "It's really difficult to talk right now as we have to get to school and I'm feeling stressed, but I can hear this is important to you. Can we talk about this tonight after dinner when I have more time to listen properly?" Make sure you prioritize this time, as going forward your child will trust you when you say this. They will recognize it's not an attempt to shut down the conversation, but an attempt to protect the conversation.

If the conversation hasn't been started and you or your child want to talk about something important, *ask the person if they have time to talk or schedule a time to talk*—"I would like to talk about something. Do you have time now or is there a better time later?"

Finding a more conducive time to have this conversation is a priority. Often there are predictable, calmer moments, so look into when there are minimal distractions or interruptions for your family. If you're feeling totally overwhelmed, remember there are other important adults in your child's life who may be able to have these soothing conversations. Don't be afraid to ask for their help.

What striking while the iron is cold looks like for Clara

Striking while the iron is HOT

I asked Clara about a recent argument with her mom. She explained she had wanted to ask if she could go to a party with friends. We went through the below questions about the specific situation.

What was Mom's mood in that moment/what was Clara's mood?
Clara said her mom had just got in from work and was trying to get dinner started. Mom was probably tired and hungry. Clara felt agitated as she was wanting to go to the party but anxious she wouldn't have her best friend to hang out with there.

How distracted was Mom/how distracted was Clara?
Mom was definitely distracted by making dinner. Clara was very focused on getting what she wanted out of her mom.

Was there enough time to talk the issue through?
Clara was going out to work so she only had five minutes to have the conversation with her mom.

Was it a private enough space?
No. Clara's sister was in the kitchen and was adding to the emotions as she kept saying if Clara was going to a party, then she should be allowed to as well. This was distracting her mom and making Clara angry.

Striking while the iron is COLD

Clara and I thought if she was going to strike while the iron was cold, how she might have done things differently. Clara recognized that if she wanted the best outcome out of this conversation, both she and her mom needed to be in a more relaxed state. Clara worked out she could have said, "Mom, I've got something I would appreciate talking to you about. Is it a good time to talk now or is there a better time later?"

Mom was also part of the session, and agreed this would have helped. However, she also recognized that if Clara had started the conversation and noticed that she or her mom were getting upset, she could have asked to pause the conversation, explaining, "I'm feeling quite stressed right now and I would like some time to calm down and think about this properly. I hear this is an important conversation, so would it work for you if we could talk about it after dinner and when you're home from work?"

Take a look at the activity below. Think of a situation when you might have had a disagreement or argument with your young person—then go through the questions in Clara's story above. Would it have been helpful to have found a better time to have the conversation?

✏️

ACTIVITY BOX

Write down when and where works well for you and your child to have good conversations. Try to schedule conversations for these settings.	Write down the situations that do not help you or your child have good conversations. Try to pause conversations in these settings.

---

2 *"I" statements*

Starting a sentence with "I" rather than "You" can revolutionize a conversation. "I" statements are typically used to explain how you might be feeling to another person. When we start a sentence with "You," this often sets up a blaming tone, putting the other person in defense mode and stopping them from listening. Also, if you're describing how you're feeling, no one can dispute this, as it's unique to your experience. Often the way we talk to our children can make them think we're angry with them when we're actually worried or sad. For example, if I said to my daughter, "I feel sad when you won't come out of your room; I worry you'll be feeling lonely. Is there anything I can do to help?," this starts a very different conversation than, "You haven't come out of your room again, you haven't got dressed, you slammed the door, what's wrong with you?"

Our "I" statement needs to be proportionate to the situation so we don't overwhelm our young person and make them feel defensive because they think we're trying to make them feel guilty, e.g., "I feel devastated that you don't want to spend time with me this weekend, it's so hurtful to me." Instead, starting with a positive statement can also help show that you want to understand how they feel, like, "I know how much you want to meet with your friends this weekend and that is important to you, but I'm feeling sad I won't get to see you." This way, you open up the conversation for thinking together and collaborative problem-solving. By doing this, your young person might go on to suggest they speak to you on the phone or meet you for a briefer period of time.

What "I" statements look like for Clara

Clara and her mom notice they quite often fall into using "You" statements when they argue. We consider a recent example together.

Mom: "You never do as I tell you!"

Clara: "But why should I? *You* never listen to me. *You* always ignore me when I'm talking!"

We explored how we could use alternative "I" statements in this scenario.

Clara: "*I* feel upset when you ignore me when *I'm* talking to you. It seems like you don't care about what *I'm* saying."

Mom: "*I* feel sad that you feel *I* don't listen to you properly."

Clara and her mom agreed that starting with "I" statements provided a feeling that they were both listening to one another and meant they could have more genuine conversations.

❸ Be specific

When we're feeling annoyed we might overgeneralize by making all-or-nothing statements—like "always" or "never." If we direct this at others, it is likely to make the other person feel awful and less likely to bring about a collaborative conversation. It's much more helpful to focus on being specific, providing an example of a recent event, rather than things that have happened over months and years. For example, "I noticed you forgot to put your bike away in the shed last night; it's a shame as it will get damaged in the rain," rather than, "You always forget to put your bike away; you've never looked after your things."

If a young person is struggling with low mood, it can make it hard to think clearly. They are more likely to get sucked into negative thought patterns, which can lead to overgeneralizing and catastrophizing. In discussions, by being specific about what might be driving the current difficult feelings, we can help our children find a clear example of what's bothering them. Having a more collaborative conversation will help them to understand that the difficulty isn't as broad as they thought. After validating the difficulty your child might be experiencing, they're more likely to accept support with any problem-solving or action which might remedy the difficulty and correct their thinking error.

What being specific looks like for Clara

Clara's sister borrowed her makeup without asking this week and they ended up arguing.

Clara: "You always take my makeup, then I can't find it. You're never considerate of me!"

Sister: "I don't *always* take your makeup. That's not true!"

Clara came up with an alternative to starting this conversation with her sister by being more specific and using an "I" statement:

Clara: "I'm frustrated that on two occasions this week you've taken my mascara without asking me."

Sister: "You're right, I love that mascara. I've only used it twice. I can see why you would be upset—I'll ask next time."

Clara was able to reflect that if her sister responded in this way, she would be inclined to share her makeup if she asked.

Clara had another example where she might have needed help from her mom to be specific.

Clara: "I'm so fed up. Everything is going wrong; I just feel like giving up."

Mom: "Oh no, that sounds terrible, poor you. Tell me more. What has happened today that has upset you so much?"

Clara: "Anabel has bailed on me again. We were supposed to go to the cinema on Friday and now she's going with Will instead. I hate feeling left out!"

Mom: "Oh dear, that is annoying; I can see why you would feel hurt and let down. . . . I wonder how you could handle this so you don't feel lonely on Friday night and you can kindly let Anabel know how much this has hurt your feelings?"

4 Put yourself in their shoes

Understanding someone else's point of view, and expressing this to them, can make it easier to have a collaborative conversation and avoid an argument. As a parent, this can sometimes feel awkward as we may worry that by doing this, it implies we fully endorse their perspective. Tuning into someone else's point of view can be difficult and requires full use of our upstairs (thinking) brain. We have to imagine what it might be like for the other person; it's likely we can only do this when we're calm and our upstairs and downstairs brain are connected. For some children, depending on their age and whether they're neurodivergent (e.g., autism, ADHD), thinking about how the other person is thinking or feeling might be a very difficult task.

To put yourself in someone else's shoes and effectively communicate this with them, you have to firstly, imagine how they might feel, and secondly, find a way of explaining to them that you are trying to understand how they might be feeling. Having done this, you can then share your own feelings.

For example, "Dad, I get that you feel angry when I don't come down for dinner when you call, but I feel frustrated when I am right in the middle of something and you expect me to drop it immediately."

When we're particularly worried about our children, thinking about how they feel can sometimes help us connect with them. Other times, it might stir up big feelings, leading us to catastrophize in our own thoughts, which can move us toward feeling overwhelmed and overreacting. Ensuring we have the right support and also approach these conversations in the time we're best resourced can help give us some distance to be more balanced in our perspective and response to others.

What putting yourself in their shoes looks like for Clara

Clara has tried to talk to Anabel about spending time with Will instead of her. It didn't go well:

Clara: "It's unfair and out of order when you leave me out and change our plans so you can be with Will."

Anabel: "Will is my boyfriend, Clara, what do you expect? Anyway, I don't leave you out."

Clara really doesn't want to fall out with Anabel. Putting herself in Anabel's shoes might help her approach this differently.

Clara: "It's great you and Will are so loved up. I understand it's important to spend time with him—it must be hard juggling everything. I'm missing spending time with you. I feel upset when you cancel things we had planned as I was really looking forward to being with you."

Anabel: "I didn't realize you felt upset. I'm sorry. I kind of take our friendship for granted a bit, as I know you'll always be there for me.

I'll try to make sure I don't do that again. Shall we meet on Saturday instead as I canceled the cinema?"

Clara and Anabel were able to share their feelings with each other, listen, and then come up with some solutions to help resolve the situation.

5 *Have a few solutions in mind*

When we go into a discussion knowing we want something but may not get our own way, it's worth going into the conversation having prepared some alternative solutions that might help overcome the difficulty. Teaching our children to be flexible and adaptive, without compromising on non-negotiables (e.g., staying safe), is an important skill to learn. Having a few solutions in your back pocket before you go into a discussion enables you to show you're willing to compromise so you don't get stuck in a stalemate situation, which could lead to an escalation in conflict: give to get.

As parents, we might have quite strong fixed ideas or expectations about what our young person should do, compared to what we might have done when we were younger, but quite often we might have to reassess some of those values we have in light of the world contexts our young people are growing up in and ensure our boundaries are proportionate to their developmental age (e.g., a seventeen-year-old wanting to go to an unsupervised party where you guess alcohol may be present compared to a fourteen-year-old in the same scenario). With the seventeen-year-old, you might not like the idea of them going to the party, but your compromise to them going could be you'll pick them up from the party at 1 a.m. (which again might be later than you would like). However, with the fourteen-year-old you may be clear they do not have your permission to go to the party, but you'll be willing to have a small group of friends over for a sleepover on another weekend.

What having a few solutions in mind looks like for Clara

Clara wanted to go to a party at a friend's whom her mom did not know. The parent would be present at the party but Clara wasn't sure her mom would let her go as she had once gone to a party before where the parents had let the partygoers drink alcohol and smoke weed and Clara had come home very ill as she was drunk. Clara needed to have this conversation at the right time for her mom (strike while the iron is cold), ensure she used "I" statements, put herself in her mom's shoes and be specific ("I feel really excited about going to this party, but I get you might be worried because last time I went to a party I drank and was sick afterward, which I know really upset you").

Clara worked out some solutions and areas where she could compromise, so she could give to get:

* Sharing the contact details of the friend's mom who was hosting the party so her mom could reach out and check the arrangements.

* Stay overnight with Anabel, whose mom was collecting her at midnight (Clara's mom trusts Anabel's mom) rather than staying at the party all night.

* Being honest about whether she would drink alcohol or not, either committing to not drinking, or only having one or two.

* Texting her mom at points in the evening so that she knew Clara was holding her in mind and being sensible.

6 Don't give up

As a parent or a young person, changing the way we interact with others can be challenging, particularly if those we're trying to build positive relationships with are not responsive to our attempts. Often when we try a new way of communicating, initially we might not get the positive response we hoped for. Old habits of interacting die hard.

However, if we persevere with applying the principles in chapter 5 (notice, connect, validate, collaborate) and these six communication hacks, we should begin to see our communication with our children become healthier and more productive.

No matter what age you are, it's possible to learn new ways of communicating with others. Our children seeing us work on developing these skills can help them learn how to resolve interpersonal problems. Many young people I work with say they overreact or push their parents away, but they're often sitting in their rooms waiting for their parents to reach out.

Even if you go into your child's room and they still seem unhappy to see you, applying the **GIVE** principles earlier in this chapter and ensuring that your child understands you're waiting to provide support keeps the door open for them to talk with you when it's a good time for them. When my daughter pushes me away, I still pop my head round her door last thing at night to say goodnight and I love her. Her grunt in reply often makes me feel sad and rejected, but I recognize that her feeling I'm still there for her despite her attempts to distance herself, is valuable. Keeping that sense of availability, even if your young person has slammed the door for the tenth time, is really important. Don't give up on making the right sort of attempts to connect with them.

Remember, young people don't respond well to direct questions like "What's wrong with you?" or "Why are you doing this?" Often, they don't know how to answer, as they don't know how to express how they're feeling and sometimes can't make sense of their own behaviors. Therefore these questions can actually be unhelpful and give the impression that we're judging them and disapproving. Curiosity and the principles in part 2 are critical to supporting the time we have with our children, both when they're younger and adolescents. Even as adults, they will still need to turn to us for support, advice, and guidance as they go on to navigate the challenges of relationships and potentially becoming parents themselves.

A quick summary of the IPT–ASD six communication skills

Strike while the iron is cold

Avoid having tricky conversations when people are in a reactive state—it's so much better to step away and take time to calm down.

Start with "I . . .," not "You . . ."

Say how YOU feel about what's happening, i.e., "I feel sad when . . ."

Be specific

Avoid all-or-nothing statements like "You always . . ." and "You never . . ." Instead, be more specific about your observation (both if it's negative and positive).

Put yourself in their shoes

Be curious about what the feeling is beneath the expression and the original intention.

Have a few solutions in mind

If you can come up with a few compromises in advance of a discussion, you'll have more opportunities to move a situation forward.

Don't give up

It's hard to keep going when your attempts to converse with your children are rejected. Be brave and try new ways of communicating to find what works for you and your child.

SUMMARY

→ The quality of our children's relationships has a big impact on their wellbeing.

→ Our child's mood is influenced by how things are going in their relationships.

→ How well things are going in our child's relationships is influenced by their mood.

→ Emotions, including low mood, can make it hard to communicate.

→ Learning key communication skills can support how we communicate with our children and in turn their wellbeing.

→ Being careful about how we say things is important (tone of voice, nonverbal body language).

→ We can improve our relationships with our children through learning to use six communication skills: striking while the iron is cold, "I" statements, be specific, put yourself in their shoes, have a few solutions in mind, and don't give up.

→ If our children learn these skills by observing us using them, they will be better equipped to manage difficulties in their relationships.

Chapter 14

Adolescence—a time of risk and opportunity

In western society, adolescence (the period from around ten to twenty-four years) represents the transition from childhood to adulthood. During this time, young people encounter many physical, emotional, cognitive and social changes that prepare them for independence. Although this concept has only developed over the last century, the historical descriptions of young people transitioning from childhood to adulthood are strikingly similar to society's current stereotypical view of them—"risk-taking, sensation-seeking and rebelling against authority" being consistent themes.[68] Understanding the uniqueness of the adolescent body–mind might explain the behaviors that have intrigued neuroscientists over recent years. With 75 percent of mental health difficulties in adulthood starting before the age of twenty-four and an increase in the number of young people presenting with challenges with their wellbeing, experiences in adolescence (good and bad) can have a big impact on what happens in the years to follow.

In this chapter, we'll explore some of the changes that occur during adolescence which impact emotional regulation and how young people relate to others. Having supportive relationships is one of the biggest predictors of good wellbeing and physical health throughout life,[69] therefore the more we can do as parents to support our teenagers build strong relationships, while helping them experience the fullness of life, the better chance they have of navigating the transition into adulthood with positive mental health.

What is the goal of adolescence?

As parents, our job is to get our children safely to adulthood. We don't just want them to survive (stay alive); we want them to thrive (meet their potential). We might have aspirations as to the kind of adult we would like our child to grow into, and the lifestyle and levels of well-being we would like them to experience. We might want to protect our children from some of the difficulties we faced when we were young to avoid the pain or disadvantages we experienced, and often want for our children what we did not have ourselves.

> ### Reflection Box
>
> Close your eyes and visualize your child as an adult. Write down your hopes for them. Consider their values; with whom and how they spend their time; their quality of life (how they feel about themselves); and the role you wish to play in their adult life.

Most of us hope our children will grow into adults who:

* are self-sufficient and socially responsible;
* are able to care for themselves and others;
* find happiness and meaning in their life through their relationships and their achievements;
* make a positive contribution to their own life and to society. Some of us may hope our children will become caring parents themselves;
* are able to cope with uncertainty, challenges, and losses;
* can ask for and accept help when needed.

Over the course of childhood, we can lose sight of this goal. The journey from the protection of childhood to the full responsibility of adulthood is an enormous one which we're massively invested in and often unprepared for. In order for our children to successfully transition from childhood to adulthood, significant changes are required to take place in our children's bodies, minds, and social world. These changes co-occur and are a vital adaptation toward adulthood. However, they also create increased pressures and challenges for our children which can have a significant impact at this time of their life. They can also create challenges for us. Especially if our children have different ideas about the kind of adult they would like to be (which does not fit with your visualization earlier) or they make different choices than we would around what they find meaning and happiness in. Ironically, they may turn toward the things we have worked hard to protect them from, and away from the life we have afforded them. This can be exceptionally painful and leave you feeling confused and concerned about what this means for your child's future.

> ☁ **Reflection Box**
>
> What stands out for you about your own adolescence? Parents I've spoken to mentioned confusion, moodiness, lie-ins, interest in sex, the importance of friendship, strong emotions (high and low), rebellion, loneliness, anxiety, body changes, peer pressure, wanting to fit in and wanting to be different. Now write down what you needed from those around you to help you through adolescence.

The push and pull of adolescence

I have two teenagers who are totally preoccupied with peer relationships, especially my daughter. Having been the fountain of all knowledge a few years ago, I'm now relegated to the position of knowing nothing useful in my family. Instead, my teenagers or their friends seem to know everything about anything relevant. I remember the moments when my son no longer wanted to hold my hand and my daughter wanted to walk home with her friends rather than me, when

I recognized my children's bodies had changed into those of adults and that sex was something they were capable of and likely to be interested in. As parents, these moments can feel bittersweet. On the one hand, we're grateful our children are making friends and growing toward maturity; on the other, it's painful as our bond with, and importance to them, has changed. It can feel rejecting, especially when they seem to lose interest in us, or change cherished plans in favor of doing something with friends—often with no apparent regard for our feelings.

Our children's relationships grow and become more complex during the adolescent years, which, in theory, we hope will allow them to build a network of supportive relationships. If things are going well with our adolescent, our relationship with them has the potential to become more influential. We can provide a safe base for them to explore their expanding and increasingly complicated world until they've learned enough to gain independence. We hope our strong foundation of unconditional love will enable us to remain a reliable relationship for them to turn to throughout their lives in an often demanding and unforgiving world.

That is the hope, at least. The reality is that our relationship with our teenager is likely to be tested and the way they behave and communicate during this period can lead to frustration and relationship breakdown. The preoccupation with "self" and distancing from family may leave us looking at a person we don't recognize. Frustratingly, when they're able to make their own decisions for their future, they may disregard our wisdom as parents. Instead, they may lean toward other influences that hold a magic we no longer seem to possess, like friends and social media/the online world.

Peer relationships

The transition from parental to peer influence is biologically driven and exceptionally powerful. The drive for social engagement is integral to the success of our teenagers going into adulthood. Being part of a community and maintaining social connection is a vital part of human evolution. There is safety in numbers (you're much less likely to be eaten by a lion if you're among the herd). Our teenagers need to work with their peers (learn pro-social behaviors) to establish themselves in their changing world. Doing this enables them to develop new social and relational skills and supportive relationships outside of the family home, which helps adolescents move toward establishing their own identities and tribes and becoming responsible.

This drive not only influences how and who our adolescents want to spend time with, but also influences how sensitive they are to social exclusion—for some, this can feel like a matter of life and death (as it would to a gazelle isolated from the herd and more likely to be targeted by a predator).

As parents we might feel surprised by how distressed our child is when they perceive they've been or could be excluded from their friends. What might seem like a minor disagreement with a friend or an unhealthy obsession with having the most on-trend brand of trainers or phone can lead us to discount or invalidate their feelings, which can unintentionally reinforce the distress. In the following section, we will explore some of the brain science behind these strong emotions, and look at how to encourage the healthy development of peer relationships while building our child's resilience to events which may cause them distress, but before we do, take a look at how relationships influence mental health below.

Fact Box

The drive to be part of a social group means the impact of bullying, being discriminated against, or having a sense of being different from peers (particularly relevant for young people who may identify as LGBTQIA+ or are neurodivergent) can create distress in adolescents and have a negative impact on their wellbeing.

Young people who want to spend time developing relationships might be unable to. Whether because of struggles with anxiety and low mood, difficulty making friends, or having a limited number of peers they identify with, these challenges can exacerbate feelings of isolation during adolescence. Their way of coping may be to further withdraw from peers and adults which can often amplify anxiety and low mood, reduce opportunities to build social skills and supportive relationships and increase the likelihood of this continuing into adulthood. It's imperative that young people struggling in this way get the right support (which we covered in parts 3 and 4) to help them feel a sense of belonging and connection with adults and peers, which will relieve the difficulties with anxiety, low mood, and social isolation.

The adolescent brain

Dr. Dan Siegel describes adolescence as the "period of life with the most power for courage and creativity."[70] This is when our children's brains are flexible, adaptive, and working in a way that encourages them to try new things (take risks) and feel emotions more intensely. These changes bring advantages and disadvantages to our adolescents and the adults who care about them. Understanding them helps us make sense of some of the behaviors we see in our teenagers and guides us toward encouraging the positives and protecting against the negatives.

In chapter 4, we explored the brain house as a useful way of understanding brain development. Neuroscience tells us that different parts of our brain develop at different rates. As illustrated on page 87, the downstairs (emotional) part of our brain is almost fully developed at birth. This is the part of the brain primarily responsible for our safety. It activates the fight-flight response and is driven by emotions. The upstairs (thinking) part of the brain is the control tower of the brain that helps plan, organize, make decisions, control our impulses, communicate through language and be able to think about what might be happening in other people's minds.

During the adolescent years, the downstairs (emotional) brain, which is linked to pleasure, excitement and reward, is highly sensitive and easily activated by taking risks, while the upstairs (thinking) brain matures at a slower rate, until around the age of twenty-four. These changes in the brain mean that teenagers are likely to feel emotions more intensely, make more impulsive decisions, and chase after rewarding and exciting activities even if they're risky. We may be surprised by our adolescents' capacity to discuss complex topics and vast world knowledge, compared with their irrational and impulsive decision-making. As parents, it can be frustrating and conflict with our hope for their capacity to maturely manage emotions and make decisions, as well as the general expectation that they should be given more responsibility and independence. For adolescents, it can also be frustrating as, despite their best intentions, they might still make mistakes and not live up to their own or others' expectations.

The adolescent brain is, however, ripe for learning and refining the development of skills (which is why adolescents are typically so good at learning languages, new sports, and developing musical talent). This is because the upstairs brain undergoes a dramatic fine-tuning during the adolescent phase (with synaptic pruning and myelination). In non-expert terms, this means "use it or lose it." If an adolescent regularly uses a particular knowledge or skill, the neural pathways for this will grow stronger. If they don't, the pathways will not be formed, meaning how our adolescents spend their time is particularly important in developing the aptitudes and habits they will take into adulthood. These processes encourage the development of integration in our adolescents' brains so the more opportunities a young person has to connect the upstairs and downstairs brain, the stronger the connections will grow—helping them balance thinking and feeling and giving us a greater chance to influence this through our support.

The impact of stress

Research shows that chronic stress in childhood and adolescence can impact the structure and function of the adolescent brain, which helps explain adolescents' increased vulnerability to developing mental health difficulties. Increased exposure to stress can leave a young person relying more on their downstairs brain (more threat-sensitive) and slow down the development of the upstairs brain. As described on page 222, thinking habits young people get into during adolescence (e.g., rumination) can influence the continuation of these styles of thinking as they go into adulthood. However, the increased plasticity (flexibility) of the adolescent brain means that they're also ripe for learning with the right support and guidance. Take a look at the fact box below for guidance around sleep and nutrition in relation to your adolescent's mood and energy levels.

⌁ Fact Box

Sleep difficulties in adolescence are very common, which can impact mood and energy levels. This is likely because during adolescence the circadian rhythm (the biology behind when we fall asleep and wake up) changes (see pages 28 and 152 for the link between sleep and wellbeing). Adolescents typically feel sleepy later and would, if allowed, wake up later. This biological shift in sleep pattern is tricky when the school schedule requires an early start. A teenager may not be tired enough to go to sleep at an early enough time to get the recommended eight to ten hours' sleep during the school week

(evidenced by fewer than a third of adolescents getting this).
The temptation is to catch up at the weekend with a big lie-in,
or perhaps have a nap when getting home from school.
However, these habits can be counter-productive and reinforce
difficulties getting to sleep at night. Adolescents need support
from families to understand the value of and how to achieve
good-quality sleep (see page 219 for top tips).

Teenagers need more nutrition and calories as they go through
the significant physical changes of adolescence. You may notice
a change in their food preferences, with a taste for higher fat
foods. Increases in estrogen may create stronger cravings for
sugar in girls, with them needing 33 percent more iron once
they start menstruating. Adolescents need more vitamins and
minerals for their development, so continuing with the advice
on page 29 can help ensure your child is getting what they
need nutritionally to support their health and wellbeing.

Emotions and decision-making

During adolescence, not only are our children motivated to spend more time with their peers, they're also more likely to be influenced by their emotions than rational thinking. This emotional intensity and desire to feel good drives young people to try new things, meet new people and ultimately powers their ability to explore, invest in the world and live an independent life. This brings many positives, including the energy, passion and vitality we might associate with youth.

The difficulty lies in the intensity of emotions, how they can change rapidly and take over the course of the day and leave those around them confused by these unexplainable mood swings. Emotions linked to relationships and friendships can be extreme (whether that is falling in love or falling out), which can result in impulse-driven actions. Adolescents are more prone to making decisions based on emotions (their downstairs brain), rather than logic and reasoning (their upstairs brain).

Doing novel things

Adolescents experience a much higher level of reward activation during novel and/or risky activities than either adults or children. This is because reward circuits in the brain create a drive toward new experiences by releasing high levels of dopamine—the feel-good neurochemical—when experiencing activities that involve risk, danger or pushing the boundaries. Feeling a bigger thrill when doing risky things encourages more risk-taking behaviors. On one hand, this is positive because it creates an inner motivation to try new things, encouraging independence. The downside of this is adolescents will be more likely to make decisions which bring about thrill or excitement, while downplaying the potential risks. This means they may seek immediate gratification without considering the longer-term consequences, putting them at higher risk of experimenting with substances like alcohol, nicotine and drugs (see the following Fact Box).

Although adolescents are more likely to take risks, they will avoid social risk more than any other risk (this is because of their need to be part of a peer group). This affects the decisions they make (e.g., taking the risk of joining in with drinking at a party over the risk of feeling ill the next day or getting into trouble with a parent). Research shows that adolescents are influenced more by other adolescents than by adults, which means that even if our children trust and rely on us, they may still be more influenced by what their friend wants them to do than what we want them to do. The downside of this is, if adolescents are surrounded by other adolescents (particularly those who have a negative influence) and do not have access to, or exclude, trusted adults, they may take part in more risky activities and make choices driven by peer opinion, which can have a detrimental influence on their lives.

This poses a dilemma for us as parents. We know successful peer relationships are key to our child's transition to adulthood. However, if our children are likely to be disproportionately influenced by other adolescents (who are prone to taking risks and making impulsive decisions), where does that leave our role as parents? Do we step back and let them get on with it? Do we take control and restrict their access to friends? In *Hold On to Your Kids*,[71] Drs. Gabor Maté and Gordon Neufeld explain that the best way parents can protect their adolescents as they transition to adulthood is by improving their connection and relationships with them. In this final section, we will look at how we do this effectively.

Fact Box

Studies show adolescents are more susceptible to alcohol and drug addiction than adults[72] for a number of reasons. Firstly, they're more likely to be attracted to the novelty of experimenting with these substances, especially if their friends are doing this (adolescents will drink more alcohol with other adolescents than if they're on their own). Secondly, their brains are more sensitive to the initial feel-good effect of alcohol/drugs, which in the moment lower inhibitions, give a sense of euphoria and relief from worries. This means young people exposed to higher levels of stress or adversity may be more vulnerable to using alcohol/drugs as a quick escape from their emotional difficulties. Thirdly, as their brains are still developing, regular use of alcohol/drugs can change the brain's reward circuitry, making them more dependent on these substances to feel a normal level of things being good, increasing their propensity for addiction both in adolescence and adulthood. Nicotine is a stimulant drug; e-cigarette use is increasing in teenagers, creating concerns around the ease of access for teenagers and the potential impact on their health and addiction.[73] *Alcohol and drug use increase the likelihood of risk-taking behaviors and puts adolescents at increased risk of harm, so educating our teens and providing appropriate boundaries can help them to make better decisions and be less likely to engage in risky behaviors. When our teen is in trouble, having pre-agreed with them that if they're in a difficult situation they can seek help from us without fearing consequences can be helpful.*

The role of parents: Manager to coach

Our parenting needs to adapt to accommodate the changes that come with our children becoming teenagers. This flexibility will support us in developing our parent–adolescent relationship and its positive reciprocal influence. Christine Carter[74] introduces the concept of "Manager to Coach" in her book, *The New Adolescence*. She suggests we take a managerial role in the lives of our children when they're young: organizing their day, preparing their food, choosing their clothes, planning their social diary, instructing them and deciding how and with whom they spend their time. As our children transition into adolescents, this manager role becomes impossible to maintain and is unhelpful for their development. Our children need to learn to become their own managers and therefore benefit from seeing us move from the position of manager to coach. In order to take the reins in their own life (with us in the background as coach, guiding and supporting them), they need us to be less involved in the micromanagement of their lives.

Parents can struggle to make this transition and get stuck in the role of manager, which can lead to a number of tensions. If our teenagers are pushing away from us and we fight to stay in the role as manager, we can end up with two scenarios:

* We have apparently compliant young people who are polite and agree with everything we ask them to do, but behind the scenes they're finding ways of taking control of their own life, which could include hiding their inner dilemmas and thoughts from us, increasing distress and isolation.

* We could see an outward rebellion with non-compliance, increased alliance with peer groups, and increased risk-taking behavior.

In both of these scenarios, the risk is that the relational gap between us and our child grows as they're not able to share the challenges and dilemmas they're facing. This means we miss the opportunity to support and guide them from the framework of a positive relationship.

By transitioning from manager to coach, we're supporting our children to make decisions for themselves. By encouraging them to use their emotional downstairs brain and thinking upstairs brain together, we're helping them to develop better-regulated and more integrated brains. This is a delicate and complex task because, as coach, we're emotionally invested in our children and we may witness them make decisions we don't agree with.

When we worry about our children's behaviors and actions, we might respond with more control, which can feel like hostility to our adolescent. If they feel misunderstood, they might respond by fighting back or trying to take back control through more extreme behaviors. Alternatively, we might feel overwhelmed and helpless, and withdraw from our child, avoiding dealing with the difficulties and hoping they will work it out for themselves. In these scenarios, our relationship with our teenager will become increasingly difficult—and the problems creating the tension may well escalate.

Boundaries in adolescence remain very important. The coaching position does not involve becoming an overly permissive parent who lets their child make all decisions and get away with everything. Instead, it's about creating a relationship and environment in which you're a supportive collaborator; not instructing them what to do but guiding with clear expectations; listening, not telling; and giving them space to express themselves. If we pay attention when they're articulating their views, they will feel valued and heard. From this place of warmth and boundaries, we can build connection and play a part in the "what next" for our children (see chapters 5 and 13 for communication tools that support these opportunities).

Top tips for parents talking to adolescents

1. Respect for respect

You might have noticed that your teenager resists when you're sharing information with them. They might respond by acting as if they don't value your input and give the impression that they already know everything. The changes in their body/brain mean they're more conscious of social status, so if they feel they are being spoken down to or not heard, they're likely to disengage. Adolescents are sensitive about being treated with respect, so Christine Carter suggests conversing with the utmost regard, as if they're the most important person in the world (imagine your body language, tone of voice and the content of your message). This immediately switches their brain into a more receptive and collaborative mode. It can feel counterintuitive, especially if they're being rude or difficult, but give it a try—it's surprisingly effective.

2. Don't nag. Ask, "What's your plan?"

Fed up of repeating a request over and over again? Noticed your teen only seems to respond when you've said something for the fifth time? Are they dependent on you nagging ("If Mom has asked me to get up for the fifth time, I probably need to get up")? Instead, try asking, "What's your plan?" This fosters a collaborative and problem-solving approach where they can take the lead with you supporting (e.g., "What's your plan for getting enough sleep?").

3. **Learn to fail**
Both parents and adolescents make mistakes, and things can break down in our relationship. The greatest gift we can give our children is offering an olive branch, reaching out to provide the opportunity for repair. It can be painful to see our children make decisions we know will bring despair or disappointment, but going through these experiences is part of life. Societal expectations can place high standards on children. We can help our teenagers to feel less ashamed when they get it wrong by reassuring them that making mistakes and learning from them is part of living a full and meaningful existence. From this, they will understand the importance of supportive relationships in helping them learn to fail safely and productively. If we lead by example with our children, showing them they can pick up a mistake and carry it as a burden or set it down and use it as a stepping stone to success, we give them the gift of courage and forgiveness.

Creating safe spaces

Parents are often surprised by how mature and capable their teenager seems when I'm guiding the conversation in a family session. I always explain that having respectful conversations is easier to do as a therapist than as a parent. Being a parent myself, I constantly fall into the trap of my own emotions driving my response to what my teenagers are doing and saying. My knee-jerk reaction when my daughter is complaining about a friend she has fallen out with is to say, "Well, I did warn you, I told you it would lead to trouble." Instead, in my role as coach, my message needs to be, "I'm with you, not against you." As such I have to bite my tongue and listen to her complaints. When she feels understood, that's the opportunity to ask questions that enable my daughter to start to work through some of her dilemmas about friendships in a safe space.

Our children are caught between all types of pressures, feelings and dilemmas. This could involve experimentation; exploring new, radical ideas; and expressing their individuality, among other things. As parents, we can provide a low-risk place for them to do some of the working out of these feelings and ideas. If we're in the right mindset, this is likely to be a safer space for exploration of these dilemmas than with peers who are likely to be less accepting of difference and less equipped to support our child with integrating the downstairs (emotional) and upstairs (thinking) brain.

If we're willing, and feel we have the emotional resilience to create a safe space, we may need to prepare ourselves for conversations on challenging topics that could evoke an emotional response in us and push us out of our comfort zone. We have to accept that we won't always know the right answer and we may have different views than our teenager on a topic. Our children will only be able to have constructive conversations with us if it feels like a safe place to come to, so we might need to hold in some of our own responses and focus on what they're saying. We may have to tolerate a degree of discomfort and sit with feelings of anxiety or disapproval. We might not agree with their views, and when our adolescents make different choices than we would, we might feel confused, scared, or concerned that they are going down a route we wouldn't approve of. Ensuring we have these conversations at the right time, right place, and right pace (see pages 105 and 111) equips us to manage our own internal world while supporting our child to make sense of theirs. Don't be afraid to step away from a conversation if it's getting heated or ask to reconvene at a better time to talk (remember "strike while the iron is cold"—page 267). It's important we educate our children on how to get the best out of us, so they can get better at choosing the right time to share their dilemmas.

The circle of trust

Our children need to trust the adults they have challenging conversations with, so even if we're not the best or the only person they speak to, we need to reinforce to them that we're willing and able to converse with them. We also need a strong network of supporters to help us navigate these demanding times. In evolutionary terms, it's unnatural to bring up children in isolation and historically, children were raised in communities, surrounded by other children and adults. As a parent, I would have been part of a tribe, or group of people, who my child and I could trust they could turn to for support, guidance and care. Finding ways to create the equivalent of a tribe for us and our children is important, otherwise they may rely exclusively on other adolescents.

Building a network of trusted adults in your life that your child can build supportive relationships with is vital (for you and for them). It could be trusted members of school staff, a youth worker at a club your child attends, an aunt or uncle, grandparent or friend. Finding balanced and wise adults your child can spend time with is critical to maintaining our child's connections with us and the influence of wise and invested adults. In the most precarious and stressful moments with my children, I've turned to these people to ask them to support me and my adolescents. In a crisis, this network of care helps to keep my children and I calm and encourages emotional containment as well as demonstrating to my children that it's OK to ask for help from others when you need to.

The challenge of social media: The good and the bad

Social media can create additional pressures and intrusions into young people's lives (a sense of no escape from the online world), but it can also be an avenue of support, providing access to peers or communities which a young person who might feel isolated in their identity can relate to and gain a sense of belonging.

Young people are heavily influenced by the information they get from other adolescents, which will inform the beliefs they form and the decisions they make. If they are exposed to inaccurate or biased information on social media, they may be vulnerable to using this in ways that are unhelpful for them. Supporting balance in this area is a key part we can play as parents in our role as coach (see chapter 3 for more on social media).

Routines and rituals

Routines and rituals help young people feel safe. Finding a predictable time of the day we can be emotionally available for our children can help provide more opportunities for connection and closeness. If our children learn to trust there are times of the day where they can have "pressure-free" time with us, they are more likely to engage in meaningful conversations. This might work differently for each family's circumstances. My youngest son is an early riser, so we always get a few minutes or so together first thing in the morning over breakfast and making his packed lunch. He goes to bed before me so I always slip in time before he goes to sleep. I use this space to get relaxed and curious, and encourage him to share his thoughts and perhaps do a gratitude exercise together (see page 36). My eldest child likes to prepare a late snack, so I try to hang around the kitchen at this time so we can touch base. My daughter likes her time with me to be protected very explicitly, so we agree we will watch something together that she enjoys at a particular time. This provides a low-stake, relaxed context for staying connected. By carving out this time, our children learn about us too—"I'll hold onto what's bugging me until Mom's in a good place later to listen to me, where I can talk and she won't overreact."

Spending regular and consistent time with friends and family, and including our children in these activities (whether simply sitting with adults and talking or playing games), provides more opportunities for these conversations to happen within our extended circle of trust.

Hanging out

It can be really hard as a parent when we see our young person moving away from us. Changes in our relationship mean as much as our children can fall out of love with us, we can fall out of love with them. There's a sadness in this that means we might hold onto some of the management role in a bid to stay connected to them. However, in doing this we might find that the majority of our interactions are based on us hassling them to do more or less of something. We should not be afraid to find ways to authentically spend positive time with our kids. We can endeavor to create protected time to have fun together, where the focus is on our relationship with them. We might need to learn the art of hanging out with them based on their changing interests, which requires a degree of flexibility from us.

Using our teenager's zest for adventure and desire for competition means we can get them involved with planning and doing activities together. Just putting up the badminton net in the garden, or being willing to play basketball, gives them the opportunity to both demonstrate their physical superiority and have fun as they thrash me! I'm always surprised how much the teenagers enjoy playing board games or watching a film, especially when other adults are over (Cards Against Humanity offers lots of opportunities for safe risk-taking!). Planning a walk where their skills of navigation are required can be fun, especially if it ends somewhere they are interested in. Remember, our adolescents have the power to turn the ordinary into the extraordinary if we let them—which could bring back some adventure to our own lives.

Planning activities that are good for wellbeing means you can combine time with your children with doing things that are good for your body and mind. We might have to insist they take part, or negotiate (e.g., "How about I drop you at your friend's Saturday—and you come on this walk I have planned Sunday?"). Their initial protests will usually subside if we get the activity, our attitude, and how present we are in the activity right. For example, my daughter is resistant to going on walks, but has an interest in the gym. I'm not that keen on the gym, but she needs an adult to accompany her, so this activity could give us a chance to spend more quality time together. I can use my daughter's enthusiasm and desire to try out new things in the gym (things I would never dream of—like battle ropes and jump boxes) to encourage me to have more fun when we're together. At the same time, my daughter benefits from my motivation to get us out of the house, away from our screens, and have positive time together. It's a win-win! Work out what works for you and your teenager and make a list to help you both to think outside of the box.

Roles and responsibilities

Our children depend on us financially for longer periods than ever before, which can be unhelpful for developing their sense of autonomy and independence. It can also limit the range of activities they have access to. Creating opportunities for our teenagers to have responsible roles in our household can equip them with the skills they need for adulthood and enable them to make a valuable contribution to family life. My children cook and take it in turns to make the family meal. As a single working parent, this skill and contribution has radically changed my life and the pressures I face in the evening. It also means they appreciate the effort required to cook for others! My eldest son is capable of doing things that I physically can't—his role involves supporting me with tasks in the house and garden that require strength and height. I value his help and I'm able to share my gratitude in a way that builds respect and appreciation.

Finding ways to channel our adolescent's strengths, aptitudes, and desire for novelty while they contribute to the family, or socially, supports their development into balanced adults. It also frees up more time for us to spend having fun with them (e.g., if they've stacked the dishwasher or hung the washing out to dry, we might have time to watch a film with them). Supporting our adolescents to channel their energy into sports, physical activity, arts, and even part-time work encourages their learning, growth, and development. Take a look at the activity below on how to create safe spaces to build stronger positive relationships.

ACTIVITY BOX

Think about your adolescent. For each of the four areas mentioned below, consider the questions and write down things you can do to create more opportunities for safe spaces to encourage supportive relationships.

Circle of trust	Think about people you trust (e.g., family/friends/professionals). How can you practically provide more opportunities for your child to spend time with them? What messages can you give to your child to encourage them to view them as trusted adults?
Routines and rituals	Think about your family's daily routines. When are you best resourced to be available to your child? Write down a time in the day you could commit to being available to your child that you think will also work for them. Have a collaborative conversation with your teen if you need to work it out together.
Hanging out	Think about the activities your teen enjoys. Try to build in time to do these activities together with you relaxing and having fun rather than instructing or hassling. Remember: give to get—getting out of your comfort zone will likely mean your teen will be more willing to get out of theirs.
Roles and responsibilities	Think about your teen's strengths and assets. How can they use these to contribute to the household? What support do they need to get going with a new role? Give them support and space. For example, if they are going to cook dinner, let them choose the meal. Meal kits are a good way to get them started. Think about what they enjoy or have an aptitude for and support them to be part of an organized group.

- -

CASE STUDY

Clara's Story (Part 2)

Clara was introduced on page 267. She's a seventeen-year-old girl struggling with low mood. With our understanding of the unique challenges of adolescence, we can go on to explore how Clara's mom might support her.

Challenge

Clara finds herself constantly wanting to be in contact with or spending time with her friends. When she's with them and things are going well, it feels better than anything else. This can create tension at home as she often feels her mom prevents her seeing her friends as much as she would want to. Clara spends a lot of time on social media watching the current trends so she can stay up-to-date with her friends. She worries that if she doesn't, her friends won't like her and she'll be excluded from the group. Sometimes when she's out with friends, she does things she isn't sure about (like drinking at a party) because it feels exciting and she's worried about not fitting in if she doesn't. Clara often feels anxious before meeting up with friends and worries that she might make a fool of herself. Sometimes she gets extremely upset when things don't go well with friends. This can happen not just when she has met up with friends, but also in response to messaging on a group chat. Thoughts about this can get stuck in her mind (rumination) and make her feel low. She doesn't turn to her mom at these times as she's worried about her reaction and that she might stop her spending time with her friends.

Clara's mom is worried about how much influence Clara's friends have on her mood and behavior. She finds it difficult to keep up with the changes in friendships and worries that Clara takes it too much to heart when things don't go to plan. Her trust in Clara has gone down since she went to a party and got so drunk she was ill afterwards. She feels Clara doesn't want to spend any time with her anymore and does not want to take any advice she might have to give. It makes her sad to feel so detached from Clara.

Opportunities

Clara's desire for social contact and validation means that if her mom can use some of the tools in this book, she has a good chance of reconnecting with her daughter and providing the support and reassurance Clara might need. Firstly, Clara's mom can think about creating situations to encourage opportunities for connection. Rather than accepting Clara staying in her room all evening most nights, she uses her GIVE skills (page 265), her mom asks if she could think about something they might be able to watch together each evening, like they used to last year. "I would really love that," Mom adds. Although Clara initially snubs this idea, her mom encourages her with the promise of her favorite snacks and a willingness to watch anything Clara wants. Clara and her mom create a new routine of watching Clara's show together at 9 p.m. Mom works hard at being fully available in this time, relaxed and interested in the show (even if it isn't her preference). In this time, she uses her connection skills (page 104) when Clara mentions something about friends, responding with kindness and curiosity to validate Clara's feelings. She starts to notice Clara sharing more. Sometimes she has to hold onto her own feelings of panic the more Clara opens up, but she has begun to learn that if she validates Clara's feelings first, she can then start to explore other ideas with her, such as solutions to some of the difficulties. If she talks to Clara with respect and without judgment, Clara seems to listen more closely to her suggestions. By putting herself in Clara's shoes and recognizing how important being accepted by her friends and doing fun things is, she gains a lot more compassion for Clara's angst and desire for excitement. Over time, Clara and her mom build an understanding that her mom can help protect Clara from herself by creating clear boundaries at times when Clara feels she cannot trust herself, such as not staying overnight at parties. Clara and her mom recognize the value of having adults to talk these dilemmas through with and help solve some of the problems that come up. Clara's aunty is fun and trustworthy so Clara's mom asks her if she can help out with dropping Clara off or collecting her from college, giving Clara regular opportunities to have another adult to talk things through with. They also decide that Clara auditioning for the college play this year would be a good idea. It would give her more focus, the opportunity to do something new and exciting and time with her drama teacher, whom she really likes. With gentle persistence from Clara's mom, a commitment to finding time to simply be together most days and not being afraid to support Clara spending time with and without her friends, Clara and her mom found their relationship grew. They discovered new things about each other and Clara learned to manage the highs and lows of adolescence with support from the adults around her, leaving her feeling a stronger sense of belonging and confidence about herself and her place in the world.

What we want our teenagers to know

As parents we can guide our children to harness their unique energy and qualities as they move into adulthood, supporting them when they struggle and encouraging them when they fail. This is not easy, and quite often, even when we are getting it right, the energy it requires from us and how challenging it is can make us feel like we are failing. It's important not to let our fear of what might go wrong hinder our relationship with our teenagers or our recognition of their individual strengths and qualities (e.g., my fear of my daughter's thirst for fun getting her into trouble can stop me enjoying this element of her character). With love for our children and all we have learned in this book, we can be the best version of ourselves—and support them to be the same.

ACTIVITY BOX

From what you've read in this chapter, what would you like to tell your adolescent? With a pen and paper, write a letter to your young person telling them what you would like them to know. It doesn't have to be a long letter, just enough to share what sometimes gets lost in our busy, daily life. For example, when I read this chapter, I want to tell my daughter: "I think you're amazing. You've the most vibrant energy, you're a force of nature, and although it doesn't always seem like it because I put in limits—which probably feels like I'm curbing your enthusiasm—I'm so proud of you. I hope you can trust me to help you find your way. I think it's important we keep spending time together. I want to learn from you because your view of the world is so refreshing and reminds me of all the possibilities there are in life. I believe you can do anything." It's up to you whether you share this with your child or not.

SUMMARY

→ The journey from childhood to adulthood involves many physical and social changes.

→ The changes that happen in our teenager's brain mean they are more influenced by friends, intense emotions, and the desire to do new and often risky activities.

→ These changes require us to adapt the way we relate to and parent our adolescent. Moving from managing toward coaching provides a presence that encourages our teenagers to turn to us for support and guidance.

→ We can build our adolescent's resilience to stress by supporting the development of positive relationships with trusted adults, through:

- building a circle of trusted adults around our children;

- creating routines and rituals that help our children reach out to us when they need assistance;

- hanging out with our children and doing activities that bring us together;

- encouraging opportunities for them to develop roles and responsibilities that build on their strengths and contribute to our household and/or society.

→ Remaining in touch with the unique and exciting energy our adolescent brings to life, and finding ways to understand and get to know them better, will help you both build a positive relationship that will last a lifetime.

Afterword

Recently, I went to see the local high school production of *High School Musical*. The audience was filled with over three hundred children, teenagers, adults, and older adults. We were all whisked into a world exploring the highs and lows of teenage life. The story is so familiar and was beautifully reenacted by the young people themselves. It told us about the pain of feeling different; the tribulations of being popular; the desire to break free from the mold of parental expectation; the excitement of new love; the hatred toward others who might be your competition; the loneliness of feeling misunderstood; the delight of unexpected alliances between different groups; and the wonder of acceptance and belonging, despite your backstory. Music, singing, and dance captured the energy and diversity of the experience of adolescence. By playing a part, these adolescents were able to clearly articulate the dilemmas of their development. The risks and opportunities.

As the play came to an end, over one hundred children stood on stage, singing their hearts out, faces beaming with joy and elation at the experience of performing and so successfully capturing their audience. I found unexpected tears streaming down my face.

These kids all looked so beautiful in their joy; so proud, so vibrant. Young people from the ages of eleven to eighteen, with so much diversity in their experiences, their physiology, their skills and talents. All with different hopes and dreams for the future. I was mindful of the complexity of each of their stories. Their childhood experiences, their families, and the wonderful mix of parents who had enabled them to get on stage and be part of this performance. Parents who had faced their own adversities and challenges. Here, working together, learning from and supporting one another to create this amazing show. Guided and led by some incredibly talented and committed adults (again, each with their own story). Every member of the young cast had to face their own vulnerability as they came on stage, supporting one another, believing in themselves, and hoping to be believed in. I could see this was an act of courage, commitment, and a powerful reminder that together, we can do great things.

My tears carried mixed emotions. A sense of rejoicing for this moment that would sit in each of these children's minds and remind them on a difficult day, "I can do great things." A feeling of gratitude for the value of community—a place where all of us, regardless of age, could come together and celebrate what each of us brings to this show of life. Finally, sadness for some of the families I've worked with where they would love to be at such a performance with their child, but can't, because they did not get the help they needed soon enough. This simple moment carried complicated feelings for me, and in turn gave the moment powerful meaning.

Learning to connect to the vulnerable parts of ourselves and the vulnerable parts of others takes courage. As you finish reading this book, I hope you've found in these pages new understanding and hope, as well as compassion for yourself, as you face one of the most complex, but rewarding roles of all: being a parent.

Further Resources

Additional support and urgent advice

If you need help for a mental health crisis, you should get expert advice. These are services available nationally. If you are experiencing an immediate emergency, please call 911.

→ **988**: Suicide and Crisis Lifeline, offering 24/7 call, text, and chat access to trained crisis counselors
→ **Substance Abuse and Mental Health Services Administration (SAMHSA)**: SAMHSA's National Helpline is a free, confidential, 24/7, 365-day-a-year treatment referral and information service for individuals and families facing mental and/or substance use disorders: **1-800-662-HELP (4357)**
→ **National Alliance on Mental Illness (NAMI) helpline: 1-800-950-NAMI (6264)** available M–F, 10 a.m.–10 p.m. ET
→ **NAMI Teen & Young Adult HelpLine: 1-800-950-6264** connects you with another young person who shares similar experiences and can offer support. *This is not a crisis line or suicide prevention line.* If you or someone you know is experiencing a crisis, call or text 988.
→ **Crisis Text Line**: provides free, 24/7, high-quality text-based mental health support and crisis intervention. Text **741741**.

Apps

There are lots of free apps available to support health and wellbeing. Here are just a few of them.

HappiMe for Young People uses four child-friendly steps to help kids unpack and understand their thoughts.

Headspace provides mindfulness tools created by experts, including meditations, sleepcasts, mindful movement, and focus exercises.

Mindshift uses CBT techniques to reduce anxiety and increase mindfulness.

myStrength creates a personalized plan that provides support for management of emotions, sleep, stress, pain, and more.

Simple Habit provides quick and easy methods of anxiety reduction for busy teens.

What's Up? utilizes both CBT and ACT methods to tackle issues such as anxiety, depression, and stress.

Woebot uses AI technology to guide 13- to 17-year-olds through engaging mental health conversations.

Books

It's All About Bodd: Helping Little Humans Manage Big Feelings—Lindy Wheeler and Tom Lawley (The Human Toolbox Company, 2019).

It's All About Bodd: Parent and Teacher Guide—Lindy Wheeler and Tom Lawley (The Human Toolbox Company, 2019).

Nodding Off: The Science of Sleep from Cradle to Grave—Alice Gregory (Bloomsbury, 2018).

Stuff that Sucks: Accepting What You Can't Change and Committing to What You Can—Ben Sedley (Robinson, 2015).

The Art of Feeling Better: How I Heal My Mental Health (and You Can Too) —Matilda Heindow (Vermillion, 2023).

Websites

aakomaproject.org focuses on the mental health and wellbeing of children and teens of color.

aap.org provides a blueprint for youth suicide prevention and signposts to safety planning tools, including a digital one at **mysafetyplan.org**.

childmind.org provides expert advice for parents of children managing a variety of behaviors.

goaskalice.columbia.edu is a Q&A resource created by Columbia University, which allows the user to ask or search for a wide variety of health-related questions, including emotional/mental health topics.

teenhelp.com offers information for both teens and parents, covering issues such as suicide, sexual abuse, and substance use.

wernative.org is a website designed by and for Indigenous teens. It provides information, resources, and ways to reach out for help.

Youngminds.org.uk have an excellent section on their website, including activity ideas to help create spaces to talk and a conversation-starter sheet called "How To Talk to Your Child About Mental Health."

Endnotes

1 Peytrignet, Sebastien, et al., "Children and young people's mental health: Covid-19 and the road ahead," The Health Foundation (2022).

2 Plewes, Joseph, "Analysis: The rise in mental health demand," *NHS Confederation* (2022).

3 "What is mental illness?" (no date), Psychiatry.org. Available at: https://www.psychiatry.org/patients-families/what-is-mental-illness (Accessed: 27 March 2023).

4 Mate, G., and Mate, D., *The myth of normal: Trauma, illness and healing in a toxic culture* (London: Vermillion, 2022).

5 Perry, B., "Bonding and attachment in maltreated children" (no date), rip.org.uk. Available at: https://fosteringandadoption.rip.org.uk/wp-content/uploads/2016/01/bonding-and-attachment-in-maltreated-children.pdf (Accessed: 28 March 2023).

6 Brady, Ann Marie, et al., "Chronic illness in childhood and early adolescence: A longitudinal exploration of co-occurring mental illness," *Development and Psychopathology,* vol. 33(3), pp. 885–98 (2021).

7 "Covid-19 pandemic triggers 25% increase in prevalence of anxiety and depression worldwide" (no date), World Health Organization. Available at: https://www.who.int/news/item/02-03-2022-covid-19-pandemic-triggers-25-increase-in-prevalence-of-anxiety-and-depression-worldwide (Accessed: 27 March 2023).

8 Aked, Jody, et al., "Five ways to wellbeing: Communicating the evidence," *New Economics Foundation* (2008).

9 Perry, "Bonding and attachment in maltreated children," p. 28.

10 Peng, Biao, et al., "Parenting style and adolescent mental health: The chain mediating effects of self-esteem and psychological inflexibility," *Frontiers in Psychology,* vol. 12 (2021).

11 "Picky eating in children" (2020), YouTube. Available at: https://www .youtube.com/watch?v=pMcxiYb4ANc&t=913s (Accessed: 27 March 2023).

12 Kabat-Zinn, J., *Wherever you go there you are: Mindfulness meditation in everyday life* (New York: Hyperion, 1994).

13 Galante, Julieta, et al., "Mindfulness-based programmes for mental health promotion in adults in nonclinical settings: A systematic review and meta-analysis of randomised controlled trials," *PLoS Medicine,* vol. 18(1), (2021).

14 Cregg, David R., and Cheavens, Jennifer S., "Healing through helping: an experimental investigation of kindness, social activities, and reappraisal as well-being interventions," *The Journal of Positive Psychology* vol. 18 (6), (2022). DOI: 10.1080/17439760.2022.2154695

15 Davies, Sally C., et al., "United Kingdom Chief Medical Officers" commentary on 'Screen-based activities and children and young people's mental health and psychosocial wellbeing: A systematic map of reviews,'" *Department of Health and Social Care* (2019).

16 Orben, Amy, and Przybylski, Andrew K., "The association between adolescent well-being and digital technology use," *Nature Human Behaviour,* vol. 3, pp. 173–82 (2019).

17 Making sense of media, "Children and parents: media use and attitudes report 2020/21," *Ofcom* (2021).

18 House of Commons Science and Technology Committee, "Impact of social media and screen-use on young people's health: Fourteenth Report of Session 2017–19," *Parliamentary Copyright House of Commons* (2019).

19 House of Commons Science and Technology Committee, p. 60.

20 Making Sense of Media, "Children and parents: media use and attitudes report 2020/21," *Ofcom* (2021).

21 Lieberman, Daniel Z., and Long, Michael E., *The molecule of more: How a single chemical in your brain drives love, sex, and creativity and will determine the fate of the human race* (Dallas: BenBella Books, 2019).

22 Granic, I., Lobel, A., and Engels, R. C. M. E., "The benefits of playing video games," *American Psychologist,* vol. 69(1), pp. 66–78 (2014). https:// doi.org/10.1037/a0034857

23 Poldrack, R., "Novelty and testing: When the brain learns and why it forgets," *Nieman Reports* (2015). Available at: https://niemanreports .org/articles/novelty-and-testing-when-the-brain-learns-and-why-it-for gets/ (Accessed: 27 March 2023).

24 Csikszentmihalyi, M., *Finding flow: The psychology of engagement with everyday life* (New York: Basic Books, 1997).

25 Siegel, D. J. and Payne Bryson, T., *The whole-brain child workbook: Practical exercises, worksheets and activities to nurture developing minds* (Wisconsin: PESI Publishing & Media, 2015).

26 Golding, K. S., "Connection before correction: Supporting parents to meet the challenges of parenting children who have been traumatised within their early parenting environments," *Children Australia*, vol. 40(2), pp. 1–8; Golding, K. S., and Hughes, D., *Creating loving attachments* (London: Jessica Kingsley, 2012); Siegel, D. J., and Payne Bryson, T., *The whole-brain child: 12 proven strategies to nurture your child's developing mind* (Robinson, 2012); Perry, B., and Szalavitz, M., *The boy who was raised as a dog* (Basic Books, 2017).

27 Siegel, D. J., *The developing mind: Toward a neurobiology of interpersonal experience* (New York: The Guildford Press, 1999).

28 Siegel, D. J. and Payne Bryson, T., p.115.

29 Golding, K. S., "Connection before correction," *Children Australia*, vol. 40(2): pp. 1–8 (2015); Golding, K. S., and Hughes, D., *Creating loving attachments: Parenting with PACE to nurture confidence and security in the troubled child* (London: Jessica Kingsley, 2012); Siegel, D. J., and Payne Bryson, T., *The Whole-brain child: 12 proven strategies to nurture your child's developing mind*; Perry, B., and Szalavitz, M., *The boy who was raised as a dog.*

30 Aldao, Amelia, et al., "Emotion-regulation strategies across psychopathology: A meta-analytic review," *Clinical Psychology Review*, vol. 30(2), pp. 217–37 (2010).

31 Golding, K., and Hughes, D. *Creating loving attachments: Parenting with PACE to nurture confidence and security in the troubled child.* (London: Jessica Kingsley Publishers, 2012).

32 Treisman, Karen, *Working with relational and developmental trauma in children and adolescents* (Abingdon: Routledge, 2016).

33 Eger, E., *The gift: 12 lessons to save your life* (London: Rider Books, 2020).

34 Brown, B., "Dare to lead list of values" (2022). Available at: https://
    brenebrown.com/resources/dare-to-lead-list-of-values/ (Accessed: 27
    March 2023).

35 Murray, L., et al., "The development of anxiety disorders in childhood:
    An integrative review," *Psychological Medicine*, vol. 39(9), pp. 1413–23
    (2009).

36 Banissy, M., *When we touch: Handshakes, hugs, high fives and the new
    science of why touch matters* (London: Orion Spring, 2023).

37 Kozlowska, Kasia, et al., *Functional somatic symptoms in children and
    adolescents: A stress-system approach to assessment and treatment,* eBook
    (Cham: Palgrave Macmillan, 2020).

38 Anderson, Elizabeth, and Shivakumar, Geetha, "Effects of exercise and
    physical activity on anxiety," *Frontiers in Psychiatry*, vol. 4 (27), (2013).

39 Kozareva, Danka A., et al., "Born this way: Hippocampal neurogenesis
    across the lifespan," *Aging Cell*, vol. 18(5), (2019).

40 Kozareva, Danka A., et al., "Born this way," p. 173.

41 Tseng, J., and Poppenk, J., "Brain meta-state transitions demarcate
    thoughts across task contexts exposing the mental noise of neuroti-
    cism," *Nat Commun* 11, 3480 (2020).

42 Tseng, J., and Poppenk, J., "Brain meta-state transitions demarcate
    thoughts across task contexts exposing the mental noise of neuroti-
    cism," p. 182.

43 Ackerman, Courtney E., "Self-fulfilling prophecy in psychology," Positive
    Psychology.com (2023). Available at: https://positivepsychology.com
    /self-fulfilling-prophecy/ (Accessed: 27 March 2023).

44 Butler, G., and Hope, T., *Managing your mind: The mental fitness guide*
    (Oxford: Oxford University Press, 2007).

45 Harris, R., *ACT made simple: An easy-to-read primer on acceptance and
    commitment therapy* (Oakland: New Harbinger Publications, Inc., 2009).

46 Pennebaker, James W., and Smyth, Joshua M., *Opening up by writing it
    down: How expressive writing improves health and eases emotional pain*
    (New York City: Guilford Publications, 2016).

47 Wood, Alex M., et al., "Gratitude and well-being: A review and theoretical
    integration," *Clinical Psychology Review*, vol. 30(7), pp. 890–905 (2010).

48 Eatough, Erin, "Learn how to start journaling. It's a ritual worth the
    time," *BetterUp* (2021).

49 Björkstrand, Johannes, et al., "Decrease in amygdala activity during
    repeated exposure to spider images predicts avoidance behavior in

spider fearful individuals," *Translational Psychiatry*, vol. 10(1), p. 292 (2020).

50 Schopf, Kathrin, et al., "The role of exposure in the treatment of anxiety in children and adolescents: Protocol of a systematic review and meta-analysis," *Systematic Reviews*, vol. 9(1), p. 96 (2020).

51 Eatough, Erin, "Learn how to start journaling," p. 222.

52 "Depressive disorder (depression)" (no date), World Health Organization. Available at: https://www.who.int/news-room/fact-sheets/detail/de pression (Accessed: 31 May 2023).

53 Moncrieff, Joanna, et al., "The serotonin theory of depression: A systematic umbrella review of the evidence," *Molecular Psychiatry*, vol. 28, (2022).

54 Bloom, Sandra L., "The sanctuary model: Developing generic inpatient programs for the treatment of psychological trauma," *Handbook of post-traumatic therapy, a practical guide to intervention, treatment, and research*, edited by Williams, Mary Beth, and Sommer, John F., Jr. (Greenwood Publishing, 1994), pp. 474–91.

55 Alsaad, Ali J., Azhar, Y., & Nasser, Y. AI. (2023). *Depression in children*. National Library of Medicine, National Institute of Health. StatPearls Publishing, 2024. https://www.ncbi.nlm.nih.gov/books/NBK534797/

56 Ilardi, Steve, *The depression cure: The six-step programme to beat depression without drugs* (London: Vermilion, 2010).

57 Siegel, Daniel J., *Brainstorm: The power and purpose of the teenage brain* (London: Scribe, 2014); Reynolds, Lauren M., and Flores, Cecilia, "Adolescent dopamine development: Connecting experience with vulnerability or resilience to psychiatric disease," *Diagnosis, management and modeling of neurodevelopmental disorders: The neuroscience of normal and pathological development*, edited by Martin, Colin R., et al. (Elsevier, 2021), pp. 295–304.

58 Roberts, Henrietta, et al., "Mechanisms of rumination change in adolescent depression (RuMeChange): Study protocol for a randomised controlled trial of rumination-focused cognitive behavioural therapy to reduce ruminative habit and risk of depressive relapse in high-ruminating adolescents," *BMC Psychiatry*, vol. 21(1), p. 206 (2021); Kujawa, Autumn, and Burkhouse, Katie L., "Vulnerability to depression in youth: Advances from affective neuroscience," *Biological Psychiatry: Cognitive Neuroscience and Neuroimaging*, vol. 2(1), pp. 28–37 (2017).

59 Plewes, Joseph, "Analysis," p. 255.

60 Lieberman, Daniel Z., and Long, Michael E., *The molecule of more*, p. 256.

61 Pass, Laura, and Reynolds, Shirley, *Brief behavioural activation for adolescent depression: A clinician's manual and session-by-session guide* (Philadelphia: Jessica Kingsley Publishers, 2020).

62 Robbins, M., *The 5 second rule*: *The fastest way to change your life* (New York: Post Hill Press, 2017).

63 Morgan, Catharine, et al., "Incidence, clinical management, and mortality risk following self harm among children and adolescents: Cohort study in primary care," *British Medical Journal (Clinical Research Ed.)*, vol. 359, (2017).

64 Kuehn, Kevin S., et al., "A meta-analysis on the affect regulation function of real-time self-injurious thoughts and behaviours," *Nature Human Behaviour*, vol. 6(7), pp. 964–74 (2022).

65 Rathus, Jill H., and Miller, Alec L., *DBT Skills Manual for Adolescents* (New York City: Guilford Publications, 2014).

66 Young, J. F., Mufson, L., and Schueler, C. M., *Preventing adolescent depression: Interpersonal Psychotherapy—adolescent skills training* (Oxford University Press, 2016).

67 Young, J. F., Mufson, L., and Schueler, C. M., *Preventing adolescent depression*, p. 299.

68 Leppanen, Luke I., "The changing perspective on adolescence," *Conspectus Borealis*, vol. 6(1), (2020).

69 "Health-related quality of life (HRQOL): Well-being concepts," *Centers for Disease Control and Prevention*.

70 Siegel, D. J., *Brainstorm*.

71 Neufeld, Gordon, and Maté, Gabor, *Hold on to your kids: Why parents need to matter more than peers* (London: Vermilion, 2019).

72 Bava, Sunita, and Tapert, Susan F., "Adolescent brain development and the risk for alcohol and other drug problems," *Neuropsychology Review*, vol. 20(4), pp. 398–413 (2010).

73 Eardley, Frank, "Vaping among teens: A growing trend?," *House of Lords Library* (2022).

74 Carter, Christine, *The new adolescence: Raising happy and successful teens in an age of anxiety and distraction* (Dallas: BenBella Books, 2020).

Acknowledgments

I had an idea to write a book. I thought, *I can make it happen*. I did. But it is not "I" but "we." It's impossible to fully acknowledge and thank everyone who has contributed to my writing of *Happy Families*. It is a lifetime of experience, learning, and believing in possibilities. Trying and failing. Adapting and succeeding. Being afraid. Being brave. And most importantly, not being alone.

First and foremost, I thank my family (both Patersons and Mosleys) for all the uniqueness they bring! In particular, my three wonderful children, who have brought peace and chaos into my life but who I would never be without. I care most deeply about them, more than anything else in the world. Without them, I would not have been able to write this book from the heart, as I have. Throughout the book, I have included glimpses into their inner world, and I thank them for letting me share these vulnerabilities for the benefit of the reader. My parents and siblings have contributed to who I am and continue to be; thank you for your support.

Next are my cheerleaders, of whom I am fortunate to have many. My beloved and honest friends have helped me on this journey, as well as the journey of life and parenthood.

I am privileged to have met and worked with many young people and their parents over the years. They have taught me so much about life and love, about pain and courage. They are why I do this work, and why I wrote this book. They inspire and motivate me, and they give me hope in the human spirit. They show me how important family is.

Over the years, key people have supported me in my endeavor to support young people's mental health. There are so many that I cannot mention them all, but I wanted to thank these individually: Dawn and Helen at the school that let me spread my wings; my Psychology in Schools Team—who have made possible so many ideas—and made such a difference to so many lives (including mine); Hannah Tuckwell at the Nest, my guardian angel (you know who you are); and importantly, the NHS, which has supported me on many levels to develop and grow and make a lasting contribution to children's mental health.

This book contains so many ideas and theories that I have learned and internalized over the last twenty-odd years of my career. I thank all these incredible researchers, theorists, and clinicians who have contributed to the field and whose ideas are woven into how I make sense of the world and others. I have not been able to name or reference them all, but for those I have, I hope I have not misrepresented their ideas.

Thank you to my literary agent, Laura Macdougall and the team at United Agents, who were quick to believe in my idea and help make it a reality. Thank you to my editor, Mireille Harper, with whom it has been a pleasure working so closely, helping me unfold my aptitude for writing at pace! It has also been a joy to work with the incredible team at Bluebird, who have been as passionate about sharing this book with others as I am and, most importantly, have the expertise to do it! Thanks also to Vimbai Shire and Victoria Godden for your brilliant copyediting and proofreading work. Thank you to Caroline Friend for her incredible support and talents with the audiobook. It was a very meaningful experience.

Finally, Chris, you happen to have only been in my life since I began to write this book, but you have been a steady and supportive presence with incredible patience. Your inspiration for the illustrations has been an unexpected contribution that has helped bring the book to life. Thank you.

Index

Page numbers in italics refer to figures and tables.

neurodevelopmental diversity
and, 284–85; pro-social
behaviors and, 284
perfection: parenting pressure on, 5;
screen time and pursuit of,
58–61; social media and pursuit
of, 58–61; unrealistic
expectations of, 58
Perry, Bruce: on attachment
importance, 27; on connection
before correction, 100
physical abuse, 18, 247
physical activity, 26, *37*, 48; example
of, *41*, 44; for mental wellbeing,
28; protection of times of day
for, 63; screen time and, 62–64;
smart watches to track, 64, 77;
Wellbeing Abacus on low mood
and, 218
physical exercise: apps to track, 77;
brain activity from, 156;
neurochemicals release from,
145
physical sensations: of anxiety, 140,
141; of worry, 164
physiological (autonomic nervous)
system: downstairs brain link to,
86–87; positive connections
support to, 26
Poldrack, Russell, 68
positive attributes, of worry, 164
positive connections, *37*, 40, 43, 48;
adverse childhood experiences
impacted by, 27; emotional
warmth, acceptance and
availability in, 27; for mental
wellbeing, 26–28; physiological
support from, 26; psychological
support from, 26; reflection box

on encouragement of, 62; social
support from, 26
power: of doing what is feared,
191–93; of relaxation response
breathing, 154–56; in relaxation
response practice, 158, 162; of
rewards, 228–29; of sorry, in
connection before correction,
110
practice: activity box on help to
build, 160; external rewards for,
160, 162; habits to help with,
159; power in relaxation
response, 158, 162
prefrontal cortex. *See* upstairs brain
preparation help, worry myth on, 172
problem-solving mistake, of parents,
103
pro-social behaviors, peer
relationships and, 284
Przybylski, Andrew, 55
psychological changes, with
emotions, 84
psychological flexibility, as mental
wellbeing determinant, 27
psychological inflexibility, from
parental rejection and
overprotection, 27
psychological support, from positive
relationships, 26
put self in child's shoes IPT-AST
communication hack, 273; case
study on, 274–75

reassurance seeking behavior, for
anxiety, 189; self-assurance
instead of, 200–202
recalibration, with online gaming
withdrawal, 70, 72

www.ingramcontent.com/pod-product-compliance
Lightning Source LLC
Chambersburg PA
CBHW031545260326
41914CB00002B/269